DATE DUE

Control Your Child's Asthma

Control Your Child's ASTHMA

A Breakthrough Program
for the Treatment and
Management of
Childhood Asthma

HAROLD J. FARBER, M.D.,
and MICHAEL BOYETTE

AN OWL BOOK

HENRY HOLT AND COMPANY   NEW YORK

Henry Holt and Company, LLC
Publishers since 1866
115 West 18th Street
New York, New York 10011
Henry Holt® is a registered trademark
of Henry Holt and Company, LLC.

Published in Canada by Fitzhenry & Whiteside Ltd.,
195 Allstate Parkway, Markham, Ontario L3R 4T8.

Library of Congress Cataloging-in-Publication Data

Farber, Harold J.
    Control your child's asthma: a breakthrough program
  for the treatment and management of childhood asthma /
  Harold J. Farber and Michael Boyette.—1st. ed.
        p. cm.
    "An Owl book."
    Includes bibliographical references and index.
    ISBN 0-8050-6455-9 (pbk.)
    1. Asthma in children—Popular works. I. Boyette, Michael. II. Title.

RJ436.A8 F37 2001
618.92'238—dc21   00-068253

AeroChamber instruction graphic on page 147 courtesy of
Monaghan Medical Corporation. Used with permission.
Turbuhaler instruction graphics on page 150 courtesy of
AstraZeneca Pharmaceuticals. Used with permission.
Drawings on pages 12, 13, 30, 31, 33, 34, 83, 140, 141, and
142 by M. Wright-Niemann.

Henry Holt books are available for special promotions
and premiums. For details contact:
Director, Special Markets.
First Edition 2001
Designed by Victoria Hartman

Printed in the United States of America
10 9 8 7 6 5 4 3 2 1

Dedicated to my patients

and their parents

Contents

Part 3: Parents' Guide

Acknowledgments

This book would not have been possible without the effort, support, and inspiration from a large number of people. Space prevents me from thanking everyone, however, I would like to acknowledge a few people whose special efforts have helped shape this book.

Guillermo Mendoza, M.D. (allergist, consultant to the National Asthma Education and Prevention Program Expert Panel Report); Fang Lin, M.D. (allergist); James Glauber, M.D., M.P.H. (Medical Director, Pediatric Populations, Neighborhood Health Plan, Boston); Michael Newhouse, M.D. (Director Medical Affairs, Inhale Therapeutics); and Mirthia Kaufman, R.N. (pediatric asthma care manager) reviewed the manuscript and generously shared their insights.

Guillermo Mendoza, M.D., has been my inspiration and mentor. Dr. Mendoza was the first, in the late 1980s, to introduce to me the (at the time revolutionary) concept that asthma could be controlled, hospitalizations could be prevented, and that written self-management plans of the green/yellow/red zone type would be the key to achieve these goals. Dr. Mendoza has gone on to show me how simple things, like giving physicians meaningful feedback about their prescribing patterns, can improve their asthma care.

Tracy A. Lieu, M.D., M.P.H., taught me a great deal about critically evaluating research and evidence. Her encouragement and support have provided me with several wonderful opportunities to do important research into what works—and what doesn't—in asthma care delivery.

Some of medicine is learned from books, but most is taught by your patients—if you can listen. The trials they face, their successes, and their failures.

Our pediatric asthma care managers, Lynn Nichols, R.R.T., Karen Smith-Wong, P.N.P., Mirthia Kaufman, R.N., and Barbara Langham, R.N., have been valuable sources of support and inspiration to me. They are the people who have changed the lives of our most difficult to control asthmatics—and the people who have changed the culture of how we care for asthma at Kaiser Permanente in Vallejo.

Emily Khalstrom, M.D., inspired me to study pediatric lung diseases. She showed me what a caring pulmonologist could do to improve the lives of children with chronic lung diseases.

A special acknowledgment goes to my colleague Harvey Kayman, M.D. I had been very frustrated at the lack of good asthma education materials available. Though I was just in my first year out of training, one night while on call in the hospital Harvey was complaining about having to rewrite a pamphlet on asthma. He knew that I was interested in asthma and asked me if I would like to take on the task. I jumped at the opportunity.

Finally, I would like to thank my wife, Dana Camp-Farber, who inspires me, keeps me grounded, and puts up with the long hours I spend with my patients and in front of my computer, reading, researching, and writing.

Harold J. Farber, M.D.
Vallejo, California

I am grateful to the many people who have contributed, directly or indirectly, to this book, especially the staff and patients of the Kaiser Permanente Medical Center, Vallejo, who generously shared their time and experiences. They helped me gain a deeper understanding of childhood asthma. I am also grateful to the Joseph family, especially Karen,

Michael, and Rebecca, who have lived with these issues and who served as a sounding board, reality check, and reviewers of early drafts. I also thank our agent, Andy Zack, for his steady hand and wise counsel in seeing this book through to completion. And, as always, I thank my wife, Randi, for her keen judgment and insights.

Michael Boyette

How to Use This Book

One of the lessons we've learned in treating asthma is the importance of clear written instructions.

In that spirit, here are a few brief words about how this book is organized:

. . .

Part 1, "The Asthma Revolution," gives you an overview of how our understanding of asthma has changed over the last several years. This evolution is important for several reasons: It will help you understand the thinking behind our current approaches to controlling asthma, and it will help alert you to asthma treatments that are now out of date. The preventive approach to asthma that we describe in the book is well accepted among asthma experts and most practitioners; unfortunately, however, some physicians haven't kept up. Finally, it will help you explain to others—family members, friends, associates—why your child's asthma treatment may be very different from what they might have learned about asthma in the past.

Part 2, "The Three Lines of Defense," explains our approach to asthma treatment—an approach that has dramatically improved the lives of thousands of children treated at our center. It offers nuts-and-bolts descriptions of what we've found to be effective. Of course, we don't recommend that you try to put together an asthma program on your own; it's a partnership among you, your child, and your doctor.

Part 3, "Parents' Guide," offers practical advice on the variety of day-to-day issues that parents and children face—everything from how to choose an inhaler or spacer to how to work with schools, health plans, and others.

.   .   .

A word about the notes: Parents tell me that one of their biggest frustrations is having to take the doctor's word for everything and having no way to independently verify what they're being told. So we've provided extensive notes referencing medical studies and professional articles.

A few years ago, these references wouldn't have been much use to many parents. But today you can find much of this medical literature (or at least descriptions in abstracts) online at sites such as the National Library of Medicine's Grateful Med site (www.nih.igm.org) or the *New England Journal of Medicine* site (www.nejm.org). A librarian at a medical library can help you track down articles as well.

These articles tend to be pretty slow reading (even for physicians), and you certainly don't need to look them up to understand the points we're making. But the citations are there if you want to dig deeper or ask your doctor about some of these studies.

Introduction:
The Mystery Epidemic

When it comes to asthma, we are living in the best of times and the worst of times.

On the one hand, we've made tremendous strides in our understanding of this disease. We know how an asthma attack starts, how it progresses, and how to break the cycle and bring it under control. We have new drugs—powerful and safe—that have transformed the lives of people with asthma and nearly freed them of the limitations that this condition used to impose.

That's the good news.

The bad news is that despite millions of dollars of research and countless studies, the number of asthma cases in the United States is going up, not down. And, frankly, we don't know why.

For example, the prevalence of asthma in children aged five to fourteen years has risen 72 percent over the past fourteen years.[1] Today, some 7.4 percent of them—more than one in fifteen—suffers from asthma.

The increase in asthma is one of the great mysteries of modern medicine. Some of it is undoubtedly due to the fact that doctors are better at spotting asthma. In the past, many asthma cases were misdiagnosed as colds, sinus infections, allergies, and the like.

But even when you factor in better diagnoses, we're seeing a lot more asthma than there used to be.

And here's the odd thing: You'd think we'd be seeing *less*.

By and large, kids are exposed to less pollution than they used to be. We've controlled, and in some cases virtually eliminated, many childhood infections. Overall, the world is less toxic for kids than it was fifty or even twenty years ago. So why are more of them getting asthma?

The deeper you look, the stranger the evidence becomes.

For example, when the Cold War ended and Germany reunited, researchers had a great opportunity to study the effects of environment on health. West Germany was one of the most advanced nations in the world, with strong environmental laws and first-class health care. East Germany, by contrast, was an environmental nightmare, full of old and dirty factories, foul air, and a crumbling health care system. And yet researchers found far less asthma in the East than in the West.[2]

Other studies showed similar surprises. For example, asthma is virtually unknown in rural China and sub-Saharan Africa, yet those environments are full of the kinds of things that trigger severe allergy attacks, such as animal danders, dust, smoke, and pollution.

Clearly, there's something about the modern Western lifestyle that causes asthma.

We don't know what it is yet, but some intriguing theories have emerged.

Our indoor environment probably plays a role. Homes are better insulated and better sealed. That cuts down on energy waste, but it increases our exposure to smoke, dust mites, molds, and cockroach allergens in the indoor environment.

Chemicals could be a factor—both those used in home construction and those we bring into our homes. Chemicals to clean and to freshen; chemicals for painting, projects, and repairs; chemicals for personal hygiene.

Or maybe we're just *too* clean and *too* safe. We know that asthma is basically the result of an overactive immune system. One provocative theory suggests that the immune system doesn't mature properly unless it's challenged early in life—in other words, that we *need* to be exposed as infants to infections, allergens, and dirt to kick-start the immune system.

Data from a study in Tucson, Arizona, lend support to this idea. The study suggests that infants who are exposed to other children and who get more colds are less likely to have asthma later on.[3] It also suggests that in some cases, a pet in the home reduces the risk of *getting* asthma[4]—even though we know that pets usually make asthma worse if you already have it.

If it's true that asthma happens because we coddle the immune system, it puts all of us in a pretty tough spot. If the only way to prevent asthma is to expose a child to life-threatening disease, I think everyone would take the asthma. (By the way, there's no evidence to suggest that any routine childhood vaccine increases the risk of getting asthma.)

Yet these theories, if true, might contain the germ of a solution to the asthma epidemic. Perhaps there's a way to give the immune system the jolt it needs without the risks—much as a vaccine stimulates the immune system without actually causing the disease. Perhaps. We're still a long way from answers to these questions.

Some see in these statistics a call for a more "natural" approach to asthma. If modern civilization is giving children asthma, so the thinking goes, wouldn't we be better off using natural remedies instead of modern drugs to treat it?

It is not an either-or. First, the question of what *causes* asthma is entirely separate from how to *treat* asthma once it shows up. Clearly, once asthma is present, avoidance of asthma triggers (chapter 6) is the best way to improve asthma control without drugs. But this is not the whole story.

In this book, we cite many studies, all of which point to the same conclusion: *Preventive medications are the best way to control asthma symptoms and head off long-term damage to your child's lungs.*

These medications can dramatically decrease the risk for hospitalizations, emergency room visits, and death from asthma. Avoiding these medications in favor of a more "natural" approach is penny-wise and pound-foolish; in all likelihood, it only means your child will suffer needlessly and may need more medication in the long run.

The bottom line: We're still trying to figure out why there's so much asthma in the world. But when it comes to treating asthma, we've seen a dramatic revolution—not only in our center, but across the country and, indeed, the world. Our goal for this book is to help you understand that revolution and take full advantage of these advances.

Control Your Child's Asthma

PART I

The Asthma Revolution

The Attack

It seems as if the attack always comes at night.

On a weekend, with the doctor's office closed until Monday.

A small frightened child and an equally frightened parent, struggling alone in the dark against a potentially life-threatening disease.

Questions fill the mother's mind: Will it pass this time—or will I need to get everyone out of bed and rush to the emergency room? Should I give her another puff on her inhaler, or has she had too much already? Was I wrong to let her play out in the cold today? If I know it's not her fault, why am I so angry? And how will we get through the weekend when I'm so exhausted?

Monday morning, at the doctor's office: "She seems to be breathing fine," they say. The look in the doctor's eyes says more: overprotective parent . . . manipulative child.

A handful of prescriptions for drugs with strange-sounding names and confusing instructions—short-acting, long-acting. Something about steroids—aren't those supposed to be bad for you? Does anybody know what the long-term side effects are? Am I doing my child harm?

Waiting at the pharmacy. The cash register rings. Again. And again.

Back home, a phone message from the school. "She's been missing so many days, she's falling behind." And another from the boss: "We need to know when you'll be in."

Arguments at home. The same old arguments. Over who can smoke and where. The dog. The carpets. And whether it isn't all just in her head anyway.

Friends and relatives are offended by the suggestion that their house is too dusty, that she can't ride in their car if they insist on smoking while driving. The teacher still doesn't see why she can't wait until lunchtime to get her inhaler from the office.

And it's only Monday.

•   •   •

I've seen the toll asthma takes on families when they show up, worried and exhausted, in a hospital emergency room. Or when they have to fight to be taken seriously by teachers, friends, and relatives. Or when they somehow have to find a way to deal with asthma on top of all the other pressures they face in their daily lives.

For too many parents and children, asthma feels like a roller coaster without the safety bar.

But it doesn't have to be that way. Not any more.

New medications and research and new insights into why asthma occurs have sparked a revolution in asthma treatment.

It used to be that all we really could do was *react* to asthma—keep an eye on it and try to manage the symptoms when they occurred. Inevitably, though, many patients bounced from crisis to crisis.

Today, we don't have to react. With the right combination of environmental controls and newer, safer medications, we can *prevent asthma symptoms from starting*.

These new techniques don't offer a cure, in the sense that we can make the underlying disease go away for good. But they come pretty close. They offer a way to *control* your child's asthma and allow him or her to lead a normal, healthy, active life.

A good analogy is nearsightedness. Glasses or contact lenses don't cure it. But they remove the limitations that nearsighted people would otherwise face, allowing them to drive, read the blackboard in school, catch a baseball, and do just about anything else that people with 20-20 vision can do.

• • •

In our medical center—and others in the Kaiser Permanente health care system—we've been working with these new medications and techniques, and we've learned how big a difference they make.

But we've learned something else as well: They're not enough.

You can think of them as tools. But even the best tools aren't much use without the knowledge of how to use them. The new medications and tools for asthma treatment are no different. By helping parents and children learn how to use them more effectively, we've seen dramatic changes for the better among our own patients.

The other part of the equation is to put parents and children *in charge* of their own asthma care. The traditional model of health care, with the doctor making most decisions and the patient following along, isn't very effective in asthma care. A large part of our success has come from helping our patients and their families understand exactly why asthma happens and what they can do to keep it under control.

We've worked with them to apply simple, common-sense techniques to make these medications even more effective with fewer side effects. We've helped them take other steps that have reduced their need for medication. And, working together, we've come up with practical solutions for the real-world problems of asthma, such as how to get relatives and teachers to understand.

We've learned from our patients as well. We've learned about the obstacles they've faced (which are surprisingly similar from one patient to the next), about their fears and concerns, about what they have discovered that works.

This book distills those lessons. You can think of it as a sort of user's manual that helps you understand and make the most of the new advances in asthma treatment.

I can't promise a secret miracle cure for asthma. But I can offer an alternative to living from one asthma crisis to the next. With the right techniques and medications, the vast majority of kids with asthma can live full and normal lives—in control of their asthma.

The Most Important Lesson

In the chapters that follow, we'll explore all of these concepts in detail.

But first I'd like to share the most important lesson we've learned about conquering asthma:

The more you expect, the more you'll achieve.

A pamphlet published by the National Institutes of Health sums it up best: "Your Asthma Can Be Controlled: Expect Nothing Less!"

When you've been living from crisis to crisis, it's easy to get discouraged. It's easy to start believing that the medications don't work, or that your child's asthma is especially resistant. It's easy to think that what you do doesn't matter much. That kind of thinking can create a vicious cycle. When kids, parents—and yes, even doctors—set their expectations too low, they're less likely to stick with the things that can really make a difference.

So if you've felt discouraged, I urge you to take the first step right now: Set your expectations high. Don't settle.

The results will follow. You and your child deserve no less.

2

Taking Control

When ten-year-old Maricella came to our clinic for the first time, she and her parents had resigned themselves to the idea that she was destined to sit out life on the sidelines.

She was afraid to join in when others played games in the schoolyard. Friends, classmates, and teachers, alarmed by her constant wheezing and coughing, regarded her with a mixture of concern and impatience. She was the kid who was different. And she figured it would always be that way.

When I met with her parents, I could see the weariness in their eyes, too. They lived with their fear the way Maricella lived with her wheezing. Would they do something—or fail to do something—that would trigger a crisis? Could they risk upsetting her with a harsh word? What if they missed the signs of an impending attack? What if she couldn't breathe in the middle of the night while they were sleeping? What if they weren't there when Maricella needed them?

Maricella had an inhaler and used it when her breathing got bad. But as hard as she tried to do what she'd been told, she'd often end up in the doctor's office or emergency room.

She missed a lot of school because of her asthma. Her grades were suffering and she was starting to fall behind. This, too, she accepted as her lot in life.

By the time Maricella enrolled in our asthma management program, she'd pretty much given up hope. Despite her youth, she'd had a lifetime of experience with doctors and hospitals, and she was cynical beyond her years about their ability to help. Sometimes, she thought, they made it sound as though it was all her fault.

She and her parents didn't really believe me when I said we thought Maricella could get her asthma under control and keep it that way. But they were willing to try a new approach.

Now Maricella is like a new person. Her asthma is controlled. She's doing well in school. She's taken up traditional Mexican dancing and travels with her ensemble to faraway cities and towns. She enjoys being active, and is no longer afraid to go out and run.

Best of all, she smiles. She's happy with who she is and what she's accomplished.

.   .   .

How did Maricella achieve this dramatic turnaround? Did we treat her with some miracle drug we'd discovered, or a secret regimen? No—all of the doctors she'd seen in the past had the same medicines and information that we had available at our clinic.

The difference was in Maricella herself. We helped her find the confidence to *take charge* of her life. We started with small victories that built into larger ones. As she began to believe in her own ability to manage her disease, a remarkable transformation took place. She got better and stayed better.

We started by helping Maricella and her parents change their thinking about asthma. Like many, they tended to view asthma as a collection of symptoms. When the symptoms occurred, you took medicine to stop them. When they went away, the asthma was under control—until the next time.

Instead of trying to manage each crisis as it came along, we helped them find ways to prevent those crises in the first place. For example, we looked at the things that triggered her asthma, such as the allergens and irritants in her environment. We took a more aggressive approach to treating conditions that could trigger a crisis or make it worse, such as sinus infections.

Then we changed medications. We introduced long-acting preventive medications, which made her breathing tubes less sensitive to inflammation. We taught her to recognize asthma flare-ups early.

We talked with her parents about changes they could make at home that could head off attacks. Recognizing that they were facing a lot of changes, we provided a knowledgeable care manager that they could call for help and advice, and to follow up with her to make sure all was going well.

By consistently applying these principles for thousands of patients like Maricella, we've achieved some remarkable results:

- From 1993 to 1998, we reduced asthma hospitalization rates by 42 percent for children under the age of 17.
- We cut the total number of days spent in hospital by 50 percent.[1]
- From 1996 to 1998, children enrolled in our asthma care management program needed two-thirds fewer hospitalizations and emergency room visits than they had in the year before they enrolled.
- We have helped thousands of children turn their lives around. They keep their asthma in good control, recognize flare-ups early, and act—early—to get their asthma back under control. They are no longer limited by asthma. They are in control.

You can see in Maricella's story many of the concepts that have contributed to these successes:

- It's easier to prevent an asthma flare-up from starting than to go from crisis to crisis. Together, we learned how to prevent her asthma from starting in the first place.
- It's easier to reverse an asthma flare-up if you can recognize it early. Maricella learned how to monitor her own lung function and how to take prompt action.
- We learned what triggered her asthma—and how to avoid it.
- We found what other medical conditions aggravated her asthma— and treated them.
- We gave Maricella and her family hope. They learned to expect her asthma to be well controlled. Then we were able to work together as a team to keep it that way.

These are simple concepts. Master these and you can control asthma. That is what this whole book is about.

Yet I know that many of us—doctors and patients—have trouble putting these principles into action. Old habits are hard to change. Nobody likes to take medicine when they feel well. It's natural to try to avoid the most powerful medicines unless we're sure that we really need them. We tolerate a mild cough or an occasional wheeze. If running too fast brings on asthma, we slow down. We're not enthusiastic about redecorating our home—ripping up expensive carpeting, for example—just because a doctor said so.

Then how do people like Maricella and her parents do it? The short answer: a step at a time. They start with the basics—high-payoff efforts that bring big benefits. Over time, they make other changes that give them even greater control.

Equally important, they learn the *why* behind their actions. As they become more knowledgeable, they're able to make better choices and figure out how to integrate these changes into day-to-day living. Ultimately, as we've seen with Maricella, they create a lifestyle that routinely puts these principles into practice.

It all starts with knowledge—understanding how the disease affects the lungs and how we can stop it. Armed with this knowledge, patients like Maricella aren't just following a list of doctor's instructions.

That's what I hope to offer you in this book: a combination of the *how*—the best techniques we've discovered for treating asthma—as well as the *why*—a look at what makes them so effective. I want to help you make choices—how to sort through all the different medicines, devices, and machines to find the ones that fit best for you and your child.

Let's start at the beginning—with a look at where we've come from in the treatment of asthma care, and an account of the revolution that led to these new tools and techniques.

3

Welcome to the Revolution

There's never been a better time to have asthma.

Over the last dozen years, we've seen a revolution in asthma treatment: powerful new medications, with fewer side effects. Clinical studies that show us more clearly than ever how to use them to best advantage. Better diagnosis and monitoring. And, most recently, a deeper understanding of how to create a plan that kids and parents can stick with.

It's a far cry from when I first learned about asthma as a medical student.

. . .

The dean of my medical school was a respected, thoughtful, elderly man. On the first day of our orientation, he announced: "Half of what we are going to teach you is false. We just don't know which half." Seeing the changes in medicine over the last eighteen years, I've come to realize the significance of his words. And perhaps nowhere have they been truer than in the treatment of asthma.

In anatomy class, we learned the basics of lung structure. The lung looks like an upside-down tree. Air enters the body through the nose and mouth. It rounds the corner at the back of the throat to enter the windpipe (also called the trachea). The windpipe (trachea) then branches to form the bronchi. The large bronchial tubes branch out to form smaller and smaller breathing tubes, just as larger branches on a tree give way to smaller and smaller branches. When the branches get very small (twiglike) we call them bronchioles. As the smallest twigs finally yield to the leaves, the bronchioles lead to the air sacs, called alveoli.

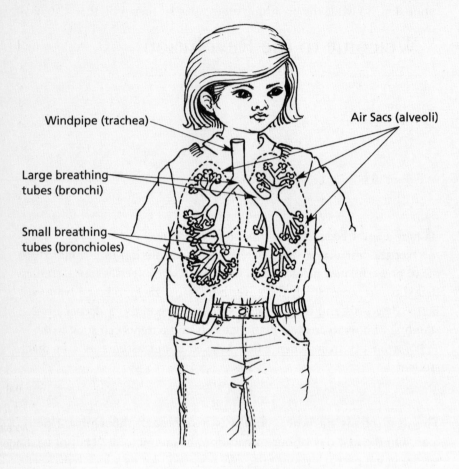

Windpipe (trachea)

Air Sacs (alveoli)

Large breathing tubes (bronchi)

Small breathing tubes (bronchioles)

Normal breathing tubes

The alveoli are where the action is. Blood from the lungs circulates through these little pockets, picking up fresh oxygen and giving off carbon dioxide. Then the heart pumps the blood throughout the body.

The whole point of inhaling is to get fresh, oxygen-laden air all the way down to the alveoli. None of this exchange takes place in the breathing tubes themselves. They simply carry the good air in and bad air out.

But these passages aren't just air-conditioning ducts. They're also a front-line defense mechanism. The lungs have more surface area in contact with the outside world than any other part of your body—including your skin. So while the breathing tubes must let the air in, they also have to keep out dirt, dust, molds, bacteria, and other harmful things.

The *lining* of the breathing tubes plays a critical role in trapping and removing these foreign substances. Most particles get trapped in the mucus that lines the mouth, nose, or breathing tubes. Small hairlike structures called *cilia* line the tubes. They're in constant motion, sort of like wheat fields on a breezy day, and gently sweep these contaminants back out toward the mouth.

Another defense mechanism is the cough. A good cough helps clear out anything that the cilia can't.

If the cilia and the cough fail to clear the contaminants, the lungs move to the next defense: inflammation. We tend to think of inflammation as a bad thing—the redness and swelling that result from a wound, for example. In fact, it's all part of the body's effort to keep itself healthy.

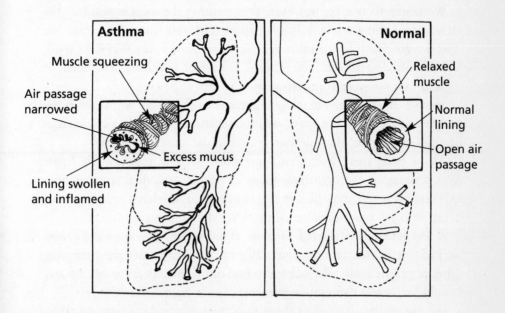

What happens to the breathing tubes in asthma

Inflammation signals the body's immune system to send in more help, and in return the body mounts a full-scale effort to drive the invaders out. For example, the symptoms of a respiratory infection—increased mucus production, a strong cough, even fever—are all signs that your body is working to fight off the offending virus or bacteria.

A muscle layer surrounds the breathing tubes (bronchioles). Inflammation of the tubes can cause this muscle layer to tighten up—kind of like a cramp.

Together, the swollen inflamed lining and the clamped-down muscle end up narrowing the breathing tubes, making it hard to breathe.

The Dean's Prophecy

In the 1980s, when I attended medical school, we thought we were close to an answer about what causes asthma. But we were looking in the wrong place. We believed that the muscle surrounding the breathing tube was the main problem.

Why did we think this? Because when we gave medicines to relax this muscle our patients felt a lot better!

We began to realize, however, that treating the muscle was not the answer to asthma control. It gave short-term relief, but long term the effects were much less promising, no matter how many ways we tried. Sometimes, despite our best efforts, a patient's asthma worsened. It seemed as if we were going from crisis to crisis.

Some even suggested maybe the answer to the riddle wasn't with the muscle at all. Maybe the *lining* was too sensitive, triggering a chain reaction (inflammation) that ultimately caused the muscle to spasm.

At the time, there were many questions but few answers. We knew from looking at the breathing tubes of people who died from asthma that there was inflammation in severe asthma. But what about in people living with mild to moderate asthma? We didn't know.[1]

A few researchers started to think about inflammation in less severe asthma. New research techniques allowed us to look into the breathing tubes of people with mild asthma to find out what was going on. Lo and behold, we saw inflammation present, even in mild asthma.[2]

Further studies started to show that corticosteroid medication taken at the start of an asthma attack could limit its severity and shorten its duration.[3] Corticosteroids are some of the most powerful medicines we have to control inflammation.

Now it looked as though we were on to something. But plenty of obstacles were still to come.

The next key event was the development of medications that could block the inflammation of the breathing tubes *and* were safe to use long term. These *inhaled* anti-inflammatory medications avoided many of the side effects of oral medications. When we tested them, we found that asthma became much better controlled, lung function improved, asthma flare-ups decreased, and our patients felt better.[4]

Experts in the field began to realize that inflammation played a central role in asthma. However, experienced generalists were slower to change. Using powerful medicines to relax the breathing tubes had worked—or had seemed to work—for more than fifty years. Why change?

Scientific progress isn't just a matter of research studies and dry presentations at meetings. It involves passion and belief—and it can get pretty emotional. People have deeply held opinions on both sides of these issues, as they should. After all, lives are at stake. The implications of treating the breathing passages were not trivial. We didn't know what kinds of drugs, if any, might be effective. We didn't know what kind of side effects might occur. And we didn't know whether they might do more harm than good.

Still, the evidence continued to accumulate. The beginning of the change came not long after, in the fall of 1991, when the National Institutes of Health convened a respected panel of asthma experts. They published the Expert Panel Report: "Guidelines for the Diagnosis and Management of Asthma."[5]

.   .   .

The next step in the revolution came when researchers started looking at the classic medications for asthma. They found that people who used lots of short-acting bronchodilators—the drugs that affected the muscle of the breathing tube—fared worse.[6] They had more hospitalizations and more emergency room visits.[7] Their risk of death from asthma was greater.[8] This was more evidence that the real culprit in asthma was inflammation, not bronchospasm. We began to realize that our primary focus in preventing and treating asthma should be on making the breathing tubes less sensitive, so that inflammation would not start up as easily.

By the mid-1990s, this view began to predominate. You might even think that would be the end of the story.

Well, not exactly.

For a while the pendulum swung too far in the opposite direction. Now you had conventional wisdom saying that the muscle didn't matter much. Specialists, encouraged by the early findings, began to use inflammation-controlling drugs more aggressively. That brought more side effects. The logic was, "If four puffs works well, then forty would work at least ten times better."

Further studies found that the inhaled steroids give most of their benefit at low to moderate doses.[9] And very high doses brought out side effects that were not seen at low to moderate doses. That was actually good news; it meant you could get most of the benefit of these drugs while avoiding most of the side effects.

The lesson? All things in moderation.

Nowadays, asthma specialists, myself included, hold the view that the inflammation of the lining of the breathing passages is the primary factor in asthma, and that's what we focus on most. But the muscle does play a role as well, and medications that can help to relax it do belong in our medical tool kit.[10]

We've just changed the emphasis. We used to rely on these symptom-relieving medicines as first line to control asthma. Now we rely on them as a second-line measure, when a moderate-dose inhaled corticosteroid doesn't provide enough control.

Research also gave us a clearer idea of the long-term implications of asthma control. We used to think of asthma as a reversible process. Yet here, too, our understanding has changed. We are learning that years of poorly controlled asthma can cause damage to the breathing tubes.[11]

Does good control of asthma with medication prevent this damage? The current research suggests that it does. Children who get their asthma into control sooner have better lung function than if asthma had been poorly controlled for several years.[12] The same thing has been found in adults—the longer their asthma has been out of control, the less the improvement that can be made.[13]

Although we are still waiting for the twenty-year follow-up studies, all of the currently available research suggests that years of poorly controlled asthma is bad for the lungs.

The Biggest Hurdle

Problem solved, right? A few puffs a day keeps the doctor away.

It should be so easy.

As effective as these asthma medications are, they are not the whole answer. Environmental factors such as smoke, strong chemicals, cockroaches, dust mites, molds, pets, and pollens play a big role.

A one-two punch worked best for most patients: By using the preventive drugs and eliminating or limiting the asthma triggers in the home environment, we could prevent most asthma attacks—and make the remaining ones much easier to manage.

But it wasn't always easy for people to make these changes. They had to undo old habits and build new ones. They had to make changes in their lifestyle as well as find ways to ensure their children took the medications even when they felt fine.

In short, we were moving from a *treatment* strategy to a *prevention* strategy. And that comes with its own set of challenges.

Prevention is sort of like the Holy Grail of medicine. Instead of treating diseases, the best strategy is to keep people from getting them. Even when we can't fix the underlying illness, we can prevent many of the consequences and complications.

But people aren't inclined to take medicine when they don't feel sick. This is particularly true for asthma, and it gets even more complicated with childhood asthma.

Naturally, parents worry about the long-term effects of medications (we'll offer a detailed look at the evidence on that issue in chapter 7), but the short answer is that the long-term risks of low to moderate doses of these long-acting medications are minimal, manageable when they do occur, and *far* less than the long-term risks of poorly controlled asthma.

Yet we still face the biggest hurdle of all: helping parents and patients create a lifestyle that incorporates these new tools and uses them effectively.

It became apparent that the best chance of beating asthma lay in helping patients to make lifestyle changes. That suggested a team approach, bringing in not just doctors, but educators, nurses, pharmacists, respiratory therapists, and others. By taking an *integrated* approach—combining medications with education and changes in the child's environment—we had a chance to put parents and patients in control.

Many others were arriving at this same conclusion. Fortunately, I had just begun an affiliation with an institution where people were putting these ideas into action, a medical care organization that had been founded on the principle of prevention.

4

An Ounce of Prevention

Back in the Great Depression, a doctor by the name of Sidney Garfield had a hospital in the southern California desert. He'd established it to care for construction workers who were building the Los Angeles Aqueduct.

As the Depression deepened, Dr. Garfield was having trouble making ends meet, and it looked as if he was going to have to close his hospital down.

Industrialist Henry Kaiser and the other contractors on the project didn't want to see the hospital close. They needed to have medical care for their workers. So they made Dr. Garfield a proposition: They would pay him five cents a day for each worker. Dr. Garfield and his hospital, in turn, would take care of workers whenever they needed medical care.

Dr. Garfield took the deal. He realized that it changed the rules. Before, he'd made money from illness and injuries. If nobody got sick or hurt, they didn't use his hospital and he didn't get paid. But under this new deal, prevention made good business sense. He got paid whether his patients were sick or well. So his patients, their employers, and his hospital would all benefit if he could figure out how to keep his patients healthy and out of the hospital.

For example, he saw that he was treating lots of workers for nail punctures, so he went out to job sites to see why. When he found that workers weren't pounding down nails flush, he persuaded the men to take a few extra whacks with the hammer to be sure the nails didn't stick up.[1]

The idea of a doctor wandering construction sites looking for hazards was pretty unorthodox in the 1930s, but it was the only way Dr. Garfield and his hospital could survive. That was really the beginning of the Kaiser Permanente health care system that I joined in 1991: a prepaid health care system with a commitment to preventive care at its foundation.

Kaiser Permanente is now the oldest and one of the largest health maintenance organizations in the United States. Today we're tackling a lot more problems than punctured feet, but the equation still holds: It's better for everyone to keep people well than to treat them when they get sick.

Asthma is a good case in point. It's the most common chronic illness of children and the most common reason for children to be hospitalized. In 1998, the medical cost of treating asthma in the United States was estimated at $7.5 billion.[2] More than half of those costs were for hospitalizations and emergency room visits.

So you can imagine that people at Kaiser Permanente were intensely interested in the new research on asthma. Just as in Dr. Garfield's day, good preventive care could keep patients out of the emergency rooms and hospitals. You can also see why physicians who were interested in these new approaches to asthma would be interested in joining Kaiser Permanente.

Guillermo Mendoza, M.D., was one of these pioneers in asthma management. He was among the first to insist that asthma could be controlled and that hospitalizations could be prevented. He said that patients should have written asthma management plans. He said that patients could monitor their own lung function to identify and respond to asthma in its early stages. He argued for a comprehensive, preventive approach to asthma care—keeping people well instead of just treating them when they got sick.

When I joined Kaiser Permanente, all these new ideas were in the air. But it took more than individual doctors, practicing on their own, to put them into effect. It took a bigger commitment.

The organization saw an opportunity to improve care and reduce costs. We expanded the asthma classes that were already in place. We started asthma clinics. We gave the doctors at each medical center feedback. We created pamphlets to educate parents and kids about the disease.

It took a while for the new research and new approaches to care to filter down to the front lines. Our patients, too, were slow to change. They were used to going from crisis to crisis, and they weren't convinced the new medications really made a difference.

But slowly, things changed. These various efforts began to evolve into a new approach to asthma care.

Our idea was to give families a complete package:

* *Medications* with a proven track record
* *Knowledge* needed to manage the disease
* *Strategies* to make lifestyle changes

We also wanted to help pediatricians do a better job of treating asthma and to provide special resources for the toughest cases. We enlisted the help of nurses, pharmacists, and respiratory therapists. We looked at how asthma was cared for in the rest of the world and incorporated the best of what we found. For example:

* We designated one physician at each medical center to be an "asthma champion"—an advocate for change.
* We assembled a pediatric asthma "best practice" team to come up with guidelines for treatment, and to monitor whether these guidelines were being followed.
* We started a pediatric asthma interest group to help spark and spread innovation.

We did research, too. For example, health services researcher Tracy Lieu, M.D., M.P.H., used data in our system to identify early warning signs that a patient might be at high risk.[3] Then we could let our doctors know who their high-risk patients were, so they could give these patients extra attention.

Dr. Mendoza came up with a simple yet powerful measure of how well doctors were treating asthma. By comparing the amount of preventive medication to the amount of quick-relief medication their patients received, he could assign a numerical score. If the doctors' patients received little preventive medication and lots of quick-relief medicine, there was a pretty good chance that these patients' asthma was not being controlled. Dr. Mendoza showed that there was a relationship between this "asthma score" and hospital admission rates. This became a powerful tool for motivating doctors.

· · ·

We also started tackling the toughest part of the challenge: working with families to make real and lasting lifestyle changes.

To make prevention work, we realized we needed to put parents and their children in charge, not the physicians. Doctors didn't live with these children's asthma the way a family did. They weren't the ones wakened in the middle of the night by a child who's having trouble breathing.

That meant bringing people like social workers, counselors, and patient-education specialists on the team—people who had the skills and knowledge to help change behavior—and we started an asthma case-management program. Patients with poorly controlled asthma were paired with a specially trained nurse or respiratory therapist.

The Kaiser Permanente "system" is really more like a loose federation, so that individual clinics and medical centers can provide care tailored to their communities' needs. Once we started making the rounds to these centers and talking about new approaches to asthma, many of them started to go even further.

All of these initiatives were like having laboratories where we could actually try out lots and lots of these new ideas. We learned from one another; we exchanged ideas. Over time, we got a sense of what made a difference.

Good news: Most of what we do revolves around simple systems and proven medications. Even patients who don't have direct access to the Kaiser Permanente programs can benefit from the lessons we've learned. Parents and children, working with their doctors, can implement these strategies. In the chapters that follow, we'll show you how.

PART II

The Three Lines of Defense

5

The Three Lines of Defense

When your child has asthma, it seems as though there's a lot to keep track of: a bunch of drugs with hard-to-pronounce names; instructions on when to use which; peak flow monitoring; the home environment; school; family issues . . . the list goes on and on.

But when you sort it all out, effective asthma treatment comes down to a pretty simple proposition: *It's far better to head off problems with asthma than to deal with them later.* That means preventing flare-ups when you can and getting on top of problems quickly when they do occur.

To accomplish those aims, we use three lines of defense against asthma:

1. **Manage the environment:** control the asthma triggers in your child's environment.
2. **Manage the breathing tubes:** make the breathing tubes less sensitive—and therefore less likely to develop asthma reactions.
3. **Manage flare-ups:** recognize asthma flare-ups early and take action to stop them before they cause big problems.

Every technique we use—and every one we discuss in this book—is aimed at one of these three elements.

If you keep in mind this idea of three lines of defense, you'll likely find it easier to see how the three work together. And you'll have a firm foundation to create and follow a self-management plan tailored to your child's needs.

We'll discuss each of these strategies in more detail later. Here's a general overview of each:

1. Managing the Environment

We start with the irritants and allergens that can set off a reaction in the lining of the breathing tubes. The cleaner the air that comes into the lungs, the less chance of triggering these responses.

Managing your environment is a powerful tool. Consider: It's completely natural. It doesn't put *any* drugs into the body. There are absolutely no side effects to worry about. And cleaner air is healthier for everyone in the family, whether they have asthma or not.

The more you can do to manage the environment on the front end, the less medication your child will need and the healthier he or she will feel.

The challenge? Many of these measures involve lifestyle changes, and that can mean some adjustments. However, we've found that these changes often seem more daunting than they are. Some are one-shot changes. Others require new habits. But after families have lived with them a while, they become second nature.

Stacks of research show where we can get the most bang for our buck when making changes in the environment. We don't have to guess. That helps us sit down with parents and outline specific strategies that will make a difference in their child's condition.

Managing the environment won't prevent every attack, but it can prevent a lot of them. And that makes a tremendous difference.

To see why, think of asthma treatment as a sort of medical bank account. The more we can prevent—and I'm talking about really truly preventing asthma, not just masking the symptoms—the less we have to draw on our bank account. That means less stress on the breathing tubes, less medication, fewer visits to the doctor's office or hospital emergency room, fewer missed days at school and, most important, a stronger sense of well-being and control.

Although measures to control the environment—at home, at school, and at work—give us a much smaller problem to work on, these can't do the job alone. In the real world, we can't lock ourselves or our children away in a perfectly controlled environment. So we'll have to turn to tools that make the lungs less sensitive to these triggers.

2. Managing the Breathing Tubes

The second line of defense is to treat the breathing tubes to make them less sensitive.

As we've seen, the medications that make the breathing tubes less sensitive fall into the broad category of anti-inflammatory medications. They block the inflammation that irritates the breathing tubes and starts the cycle of asthma. They are designed to be used each and every day to keep the breathing tubes feeling normal. Asthma experts also call them "preventive" or "long-acting controller" medicines. These preventive medicines are different from the quick-relief medicines that temporarily lessen asthma symptoms.*

The big mistake that most people make with these medicines is in thinking that they work quickly. They don't. Most take about one to two weeks before exhibiting an effect and one to two months for maximum effect. They work best when the breathing tubes are normal—that is, before a flare-up starts. Otherwise, it's like closing the barn door after the horse is out.

The biggest challenge is using the medications consistently and incorporating them into your child's daily routine. When these medications are doing their job, you don't notice them. Your child simply feels normal—and that's when the trouble starts. It's easy to become complacent. The more the asthma is under control, the less attention you pay to it. So your child may forget to take the preventive medicines, or feel he or she no longer needs it. Until the next crisis.

These drugs have an excellent track record of safety and effectiveness.

---

*A word about terminology: The two main categories of inhaled drugs are: (1) The *long-term asthma controllers* like inhaled corticosteroids. These medications, if used every day, prevent asthma inflammation from starting. They do not provide quick relief of asthma symptoms. (2) The medications that provide *quick relief* of asthma symptoms, but whose effects wear off after a few hours.

For the sake of clarity, we'll usually refer to the first as "preventive" and the second as "quick-relief."

In later chapters, we'll look more closely at the risks and benefits. We'll discuss how to find the asthma prevention strategy that meets your individual needs—with the minimum amount of medication. And we'll discuss what exists currently, and explore the exciting new medications that are in development.

3. Managing Flare-Ups

The third line of defense is to recognize flare-ups early and take aggressive action to keep them from escalating.

There's an old saying: You can't manage what you can't measure. To recognize flare-ups early, you need a way to keep score. Part of our program involves teaching kids and parents how to measure their lung function, and how to take action based on the results.

If your child has had asthma for any length of time, chances are you're familiar with the peak flow meter. A peak flow meter can measure just how tight the breathing tubes are. But we've found that it takes some training and reinforcement to be sure it's used properly. Later in the book we will discuss how to choose a peak flow meter and how to be sure you're using it right (chapter 12).

It's also important to be sensitive to the early signs and symptoms of asthma—such as a dry cough, mild wheeze, or a scratchy throat. In chapter 9 we'll discuss how to use signs and symptoms to recognize asthma severity level and determine what action needs to be taken. With good asthma control, flare-ups should be the exception, not the rule. If they do occur, they should not be as bad.

Here, too, we emphasize *early* action. The medicine works better if you start it sooner. And results in less wear and tear—psychologically as well as physically—on you and your child.

An Integrated Approach

None of these three strategies are the complete solution. One is not a "better" strategy than the others. Rather, they all work together—in three separate ways—to enable parents and kids to take control of their asthma.

It's sort of like gardening: You need fertile soil, water, and sunlight to make plants grow. You can't do it with just one of the three.

• • •

In a nutshell, this is the program: Control asthma triggers in your child's environment. Use preventive medications to make the breathing tubes less sensitive and prevent flare-ups. Take early action to keep flare-ups from getting out of hand.

In the chapters that follow, we'll discuss each component in detail. And then we'll show you how to put it all together to create a plan that best meets your individual needs.

The Tools We Use

This three-pronged approach wouldn't be possible without tools that can deliver medication directly to the breathing tubes and tools to measure lung function.

Chapter 12 offers a detailed guide to the specific devices on the market. But it's useful at this point to give you a general overview of these tools and how they work.

Getting Medicine to the Lungs

The Metered Dose Inhaler (MDI)

Most people are familiar with the little pressured canisters that deliver a puff of asthma medicine. They seem simple enough, but it's no simple task to get the right amount of medicine to the right place.

Also called MDIs, inhalers, or puffers, these are the most widely used devices to get medication into the lungs. They're called "metered-dose" inhalers because they deliver a consistent (metered) amount of medicine with each puff. With current technology, anyone from birth to old age can use a metered-dose inhaler.

The metered-dose inhaler contains medicine as well as a pressurized liquid (usually, chlorofluorocarbons or CFCs) that expands into a gas as it passes through the nozzle. This liquid, known as propellant, breaks up the medicine into a mist of fine droplets and forces it out the nozzle and (we hope) into your child's lungs.

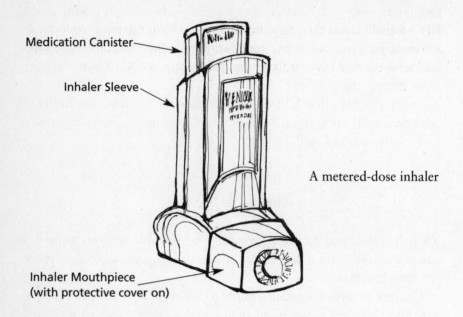

Medication Canister

Inhaler Sleeve

A metered-dose inhaler

Inhaler Mouthpiece
(with protective cover on)

But here's the rub: The lungs are designed to keep unwanted stuff out, and before the medicine can get to the breathing tubes, it has to pass through a number of barriers: the nose, the mouth, the throat, and the trachea (windpipe). Large, fast-moving particles, like fast-moving race cars, have trouble negotiating curves, such as the turn from the mouth to the throat into the windpipe.

And (continuing our car analogy) big lumbering particles do the worst of all. Like a big old Lincoln trying to take a hairpin turn, they tend to end up in the ditches on the side of the road. The large particles of medicine released from your inhaler settle in the nose, throat, windpipe, or large breathing tubes, never making it down to the small breathing tubes where the problems with asthma occur.

The challenge, then, in designing medication for inhalation is to maximize the number of small particles, minimize the number of large particles, and slow them down enough so that they can round the corners to get deeply into the lungs.

The key advantage of metered-dose inhalers is their simplicity. They're quick and convenient to use. Their disadvantages: If the correct technique isn't used, the medication may not get to the lungs. Even with the best technique, only 10 to 20 percent of a dose gets there. In addition, the CFCs found in most metered-dose inhalers are harmful to the ozone layer.

Fortunately, we have another tool that helps overcome the inefficiency of metered-dose inhalers: the spacer.

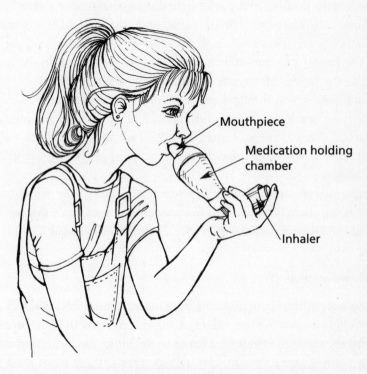

Mouthpiece

Medication holding chamber

Inhaler

Using a metered-dose inhaler via a tube-type spacer

Spacers

A spacer device, also called a "holding chamber," is a device that places some space between a metered-dose inhaler and the mouth. It can be in the form of a tube or a plastic bag. On one end, you insert the inhaler. The other end has a mouthpiece. It helps medicine from a metered-dose inhaler get into the lungs better.

I feel that metered-dose inhalers should *always* be used with a spacer device. The reason: It helps more of the medicine get to the lungs—where you need it. It helps to keep the medicine from the mouth and throat, where it does the breathing tubes no good at all. Without a spacer, you need to puff and inhale at the same time. If the coordination is less than perfect, little or no medicine may get to where you need it. A spacer holds the medication for a few seconds, so that it can be inhaled more effectively.

By briefly holding the puff of medicine, the spacer device allows the larger droplets to settle out—the ones that would never make it to the lungs anyway. The small particles (the ones that can get deep into the lungs) stay suspended. The net result: less drug in the mouth, more in the lungs; better effectiveness and fewer side effects.

Some people feel that spacers are just for kids who can't coordinate use of their inhaler and that adults should be able to use the inhaler all by itself. I don't agree with that. People of all ages should use a spacer with their metered-dose inhaler because it helps get the medicine where it belongs.

Some spacers are rather bulky, which can make kids self-conscious about using them. They're also one more thing kids have to keep track of. But the advantages far outweigh these minor drawbacks.

Dry Powder Inhalers

Dry powder inhalers are different from metered-dose inhalers. Dry powder inhalers do not use propellant. A rapid, deep breath is the force that propels the medicine from the inhaler to the lungs. Because the medicine is not coming out of the inhaler at high speed, there is no need for a spacer to slow it down.

A child needs to be old enough to take a deep, rapid breath in and hold it to use a dry powder inhaler. Generally children older than seven or eight years can understand and coordinate this.

One disadvantage of these devices is that during a severe asthma flare-up, a person may have trouble taking the fast, deep breath needed to get the medicine into the lungs.

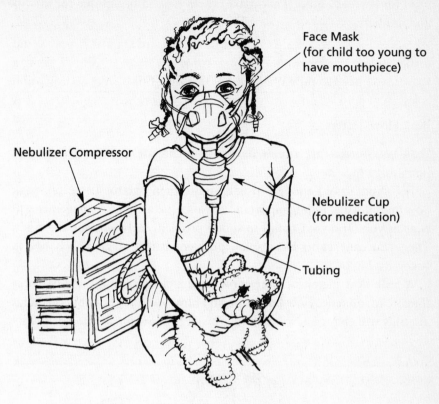

Face Mask
(for child too young to
have mouthpiece)

Nebulizer Compressor

Nebulizer Cup
(for medication)

Tubing

Using a nebulizer machine

Nebulizers

Also known as breathing treatment machines, these are electric-powdered machines that make the liquid medicine into a mist that you inhale for about 15 minutes.

Nebulizers are much less efficient in delivering medicine than inhalers. We make up for this inefficiency by loading much more medicine into the nebulizer. For example, the dose of albuterol in a metered-dose inhaler is 0.09 mg. However, in a nebulizer the usual dose is 2.5 mg—almost 30 times as much.

Though less efficient than an inhaler, nebulizers are simple to use. Pretty much all you have to do to get the medication from it is to sit there and breathe—no need to coordinate puffing and breathing, no need for a breath hold. That makes them especially suitable for infants and toddlers.

Measuring Lung Function

Peak Flow Meters

Peak flow meters are simple devices you can use at home to measure lung function.

For children old enough (usually more than five to six years), peak flow monitoring is an important advance in asthma management. It enables you (and your child) to spot a problem early—before the crisis. Then you can act to fix a small problem before it gets a chance to become a big one.

A peak flow meter measures how hard a person can blow out. Three things can influence how hard a person blows out; (1) how big the lungs are (this will change as your child grows); (2) how much effort is put in;

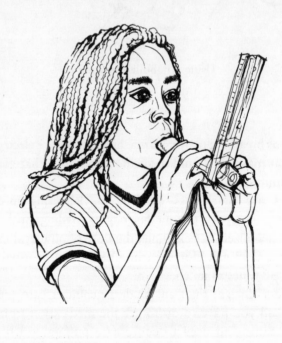

Using a peak flow meter to measure lung function

(3) how tight or open the breathing tubes are. If your child has not grown that much since you last checked, and maximal effort is being put in, then all that will alter the peak flow is how tight or open the breathing tubes are. If the peak flow rate is close to your child's personal best, then asthma is in good control. If the peak flow rate has significantly dropped from the personal best, the breathing tubes are starting to tighten. Asthma is starting to flare, and action needs to be taken.

Information from peak flow monitoring can be used to establish an asthma management plan (see chapter 9) so you know what medication to give your child for what levels of lung function. Information from peak flow monitoring can also be used to tell how well (or poorly) controlled your child's asthma is. This can let you, and your doctor, know if more aggressive action is needed, or if medications can be decreased.

6

Managing the Environment

The more we can do to manage the environment, the less we have to rely on drugs to control asthma. That means better control, less medicine, and fewer side effects.

When we look at the effects of the environment on asthma, we usually think of them in terms of *triggers*. Asthma triggers set off reactions in the breathing tubes. Smoke, dust, molds, animal dander, and pollens are all asthma triggers.

The key to managing the environment is to identify your child's triggers, eliminate or reduce them, and keep them from getting into the lungs.

What's a Trigger?

Think of the last time you got a splinter in your hand. The splinter itself may have been so small you could barely see it. But before long, the skin around it was red, swollen, and inflamed.

That's pretty much what happens in the breathing tubes of people with asthma. When the lung's defenses detect something foreign—be it a smoke particle, an allergen, or an infection—it rallies its defenses to drive it out. In people with asthma, these defenses overreact.

Asthma triggers cause the breathing tubes to become swollen and inflamed. The inflammation, in turn, makes the muscle that lines the outside of the breathing tube squeeze down. At the same time, the inflamed breathing tube starts to make mucus (much like a cold virus or allergies causing a runny nose).

As you can see, the one-two-three punch all starts with the inflammation, so a good way to control asthma is by heading off this inflammation. One of the best ways to do that is by controlling your child's exposure to asthma triggers.

Think of it this way: the fewer triggers, the less inflammation. Hence, the less need for medication, fewer crises, and less discomfort for you and your children.

The bottom line: Controlling asthma triggers is like prescribing a drug that works for everyone, is 100 percent safe, and has no dangerous side effects.

Managing the environment offers benefits for the rest of the family, too. The triggers that cause asthma in one child may well be causing trouble for others. A smoke-free home, for example, will benefit the whole family.

There are three types of asthma triggers:

- **Allergens:** Common inhaled allergens include animal dander (the shed skin of your furry or feathered pets), house dust mites, molds, cockroach droppings, and pollens. Allergy testing can tell if these are problems for your child, and how much action you need to take to control them.
- **Irritants:** These cause trouble for everyone. You don't have to be allergic. Smoke (from any source) is one of the most common irritants in our environment. Strong chemicals are another.
- **Infections:** Some are viral, like the common cold. Others can be bacterial, like a sinus infection or pneumonia. Knowing what kind of infection is important—antibiotics won't help if it is a virus.

When looking at asthma triggers, we usually focus first on those in the home. Why? Because they're the triggers that families can best control, and because most of our lives are spent at home. Within the home, we focus mostly on the bedroom, for the same reasons: About a third of our lives are spent there.

Here are some of the most common asthma triggers in the home, and some simple strategies with big payoffs.

Smoke

Smoke is an irritant, and is by far one of the most common and most potent asthma triggers. It is bad for all of us, and much more so for people with asthma. In a study of Medicaid-insured children with asthma, almost 60 percent of children lived in homes where someone smoked.[1]

During my fellowship at Tulane University in New Orleans, Louisiana, I looked into how much asthma is caused by smoking. I was amazed to find almost one-third more asthma among the children whose mothers smoked.[2]

Here's what that means: If you or someone in your family smokes, *you can dramatically improve, and possibly cure your child's asthma* just by getting smoke out of the home.

If you smoke and your child has asthma, it's worth just about anything you can do to kick the habit. Until you are able to quit, keep the smoke strictly outside. Not in the bedroom, not the bathroom, not the garage. Strictly outside. A friend of mine once joked that having a room in your home for smoking is like having one section of a swimming pool for peeing.

You may not see differences overnight. It may take days for the smoke to clear from your home. It will take longer for the inflammation of the breathing tubes to respond. The inflammation got there after years of smoke exposure; it will take a while for it to go away.

When I was living in New Orleans, my next-door neighbor told me that her daughter had asthma. Her chest would get tight with any vigorous activity. She needed lots of doctor visits. She was missing lots of school.

While we were talking, I noticed the pack of cigarettes in her pocket. I suggested, "If you could find a way to stop smoking, I bet it would help a lot with your daughter's asthma."

She didn't say much, so I was surprised three weeks later when she proudly informed me she'd quit.

"And how's your daughter?" I asked.

Her face beamed. "She's doing great!" she said.

Now, consider the impact of what she'd achieved. She'd been struggling for years to get her daughter's asthma under control. Then she'd done *one* thing—admittedly, one very big thing—that was more effective than all those earlier efforts combined. And she achieved it without having to give her daughter any more drugs!

Kicking the Habit

Quitting isn't easy. Tobacco can be as addictive as heroin, if not more so. But the first steps can be small: Get information. Make a phone call. Don't think of what it takes to quit now. Think about what it will take to get a little bit closer to quitting.

Get out a pen and paper. Write down the answers to the following: Why do you want to quit? When you tried to quit in the past, what helped and what didn't? What will be the most difficult situations for you after you quit? How will you plan to handle them? Who can help you through the tough times? Your family? Friends? Health care provider? What pleasures do you get from smoking? What ways can you still get pleasure when you quit?

Write down questions to ask your doctor, such as: How can you help me to be successful at quitting? What medication do you think would be best for me and how should I take it? What should I do if I need more help?[3]

Getting support is important. Research shows that the more support you have, the greater your chance for success in quitting. Enlist the support of family and friends. Join a stop-smoking program.

Learn how to handle the urge to smoke. Be aware of the things that may cause you to smoke, such as other smokers, stress, depression, and alcohol.[4]

Smoking helps with stress, hunger, and boredom. Find other things to play that role. Take a hot bath, exercise, meditate, read a good book.

What about medications for quitting? Talk to your doctor about what is right for you. Nicotine gum or patches help with the withdrawal symptoms. Bupropion (Zyban) is a pill available by prescription. This medicine can be very helpful in decreasing the craving.

List the things you need to do to quit. The first may be deciding that you want to quit. The second may be getting into a stop-smoking class. The third may be getting nicotine patches or a prescription for medicine to help with the craving. Enlist your family's support. Set a quit date.

Don't be discouraged if you don't succeed the first time. Some people just up and quit, but they're the exception. Most need a series of "practice runs." On each of these practice runs you learn something—about what works for you, and what doesn't. Important information that will help you succeed.

Be sure to give yourself something back as a reward for your success. Do something pleasurable every day. Sock away the money you would have spent on cigarettes and use it to buy something special. If you smoked one pack a day, after having quit for a year you will have saved enough for a vacation to Hawaii or the Caribbean! What a wonderful reward for doing something good for your children and yourself.

Other Sources of Smoke

Cigarette smoke may not be the only smoke in your home. Fireplaces, incense, and burned food are all common sources of smoke—and asthma triggers.

Many people don't think of a fireplace as a source of smoke, but it is. It can add to asthma trouble just as well as a smoker in the home. If anyone in the family has asthma, avoid using the fireplace.

Even the burning of "clean" natural gas or propane can irritate the lungs. Though you won't see a lot of soot, burning natural gas or propane liberates substances called nitrogen oxides. Nitrogen oxides can irritate the lining of the lungs, causing asthma. If you have a choice, it's better to use electricity for heating and cooking. If you do have a gas stove or heater, be sure to have good ventilation in the room.

Pets

Pets with fur or feathers can be major league sources of allergens. Many people think that dogs whose fur doesn't shed, such as terriers and poodles, won't cause allergic reactions. Not so—it's their shed skin that is the allergen, not the fur itself. For cats, add their saliva too.

Some people, especially those from Mexico, feel that Chihuahua dogs are good for asthma, which is ironic, since the dogs themselves may make a wheeze-like noise. However, if you have asthma and you're allergic to dogs, Chihuahuas are just as likely to trigger asthma as other breeds.

Dogs and cats aren't the only pets that can trigger asthma. Mice, gerbils, rabbits, hamsters, guinea pigs, and birds—anything with fur or feathers—can trigger it, too. In my experience, cat allergen tends to be one of the worst, but every individual is different.

Allergy testing can tell you if the pet is adding to your child's asthma problem (see box on page 46 for more information on allergy testing). A positive skin test is a pretty strong sign that getting the pet out the home will improve your child's asthma. It can take months for the pet allergen to clear from your home after the pet has left, so you may not see the difference right away.

This is a tough challenge for many families. When I suggest giving up the family pet, I might as well be suggesting that they sell one of the children.

Few families are willing to find a new home for Fido—at least not right away. Less drastic measures can help, but I'm going to stand my ground and say that finding a new home for your pet can be a powerful step in getting your child's asthma under control.

As you weigh the trade-offs, I urge you to keep in mind a story that one mother told me when I was in Tucson, Arizona.

Her twins had always had asthma. The children frequently slept with their pet cats. They never seemed to be allergic to them. They didn't itch or break out in hives. Their asthma didn't seem any worse or better whether they slept with the cats or not. So the parents were convinced that the cats weren't a major factor in the kids' asthma.

Finally the twins grew up and went off to college, leaving the cats at home. At college, their asthma got a lot better. It seemed as if they'd grown out of it.

But when they returned home, they started to cough and wheeze again. Now their asthma was noticeably worse when they spent time with the cats.

So what happened? Had they suddenly developed cat allergies?

The likeliest explanation: They *always* were allergic to the cats. When they lived with the cats every day they were continuously exposed to the cat allergen, so it made no difference whether the cats were near or far. But once they'd been away from the allergens for a while and their lungs had normalized, the reaction was more noticeable.

The moral of the story: Sometimes the cause-and-effect relationship isn't obvious. That's why allergy testing is important.

Sometimes, however, it's just not possible to give up a pet. So other steps become important. Keeping the pet outside is one solution. One family built a beautiful house for the cat in the front yard.

Other families may not be able to go that far. Maybe there's no yard to keep the pet in. Maybe the pet has always been indoors. Maybe the weather is too harsh. In these cases bathing the pet weekly can drastically decrease the amount of allergen they shed. Keeping the pet in the garage rather than the house may help too.

Pet allergen tends to stay in the air for long periods, so a HEPA-filtered air cleaner will help. Put one in each room where your child spends a lot of time. Be sure to have one in the bedroom. If you have central heat or air conditioning, use high-efficiency filters there as well. At an absolute minimum, be sure to keep the pet out of the bedroom.

Dust Mites

The third big offender, the dust mite, is a microscopic creature that lives in house dust. It doesn't bite and isn't otherwise harmful, but it does trigger an allergic reaction in the lungs and breathing passages.

Not in my house, you say? I'm afraid I have bad news: Dust mites live just about anywhere that you find dust and a reasonable amount of humidity. They love woven material like bedding, pillows, teddy bears, carpeting, and upholstered furniture.

I might as well tell you the rest of the bad news now. It's really their droppings that cause the allergic reaction, and your shed skin serves as their food.

Dust-mite allergens tend to settle out of the air quickly. But when you lie or sit on a dust-mite reservoir—like a bed or an upholstered couch—you unleash a whole load of allergen right into the air you are breathing. When you sleep with your face in a pillow, you're breathing in dust mite allergen all night.

The best defenses against dust mites in the bedroom are allergen-proof encasings. They create a barrier between the mattress, pillow, or cushions and your lungs.

The technology for allergen-proof encasings has improved dramatically from the crinkly plastic stuff that I grew up with. Much of what is on the market now is comfortable, soft, and breathable. See your local allergy products supplier, or the list of allergy supply firms in appendix C.

Dust mites also thrive in sheets and blankets—even in the stuffed animals your child sleeps with. Washing the bedding in hot water will help to kill them. You need very hot water—at least 140° F. Water this hot can scald, so after the laundry is done, be sure to turn the hot water temperature back down to safe levels.

Be sure to wash everything on the bed in hot water. The sheets, the blankets, the comforter, the pillowcases, even the stuffed animals. If you can't bear to wash Teddy Bear in hot water, putting it in the dryer until it gets really hot and toasty may do the job.

You can make your home unfriendly to dust mites. Hardwood or tile floors are better than carpets. Getting rid of clutter gives dust mites fewer places to hide. Vinyl or leather furniture doesn't provide the warm cozy space for the dust mites to cuddle into as an upholstered couch does. If you live in a very humid area, using a dehumidifier may help.

If you can't remove the carpeting, vacuum it weekly. Use a vacuum with a HEPA (high-efficiency particulate air) filter. The price of HEPA vacuums has come down dramatically. Though some models can cost up to $1,000, I have seen good products on the market for $150 to $200.

How do you know if you need to take all these steps? The allergy test will tell you.

Cockroaches

Cockroach allergen is a highly potent trigger of asthma. The National Inner City Asthma Study found that children who are allergic to cockroaches and who live in cockroach-infested homes are much more likely to need emergency room visits or hospitalization for their asthma. Their risk of severe asthma is that much higher.

Allergies to cockroaches are common, too. More than one-third of the children in the National Inner City Asthma Study were allergic. A high level of cockroach allergen was found in more than half of these children's bedrooms.[5]

Cockroach allergen comes from their droppings, their saliva, eggs, and shed cuticle (what passes for roach skin). Even if you don't see cockroaches, they may still be causing problems if their droppings are about. If one roach is seen, chances are that hundreds more are hidden.

Controlling cockroaches is difficult. Once they've established themselves in your home or apartment it is tough to get rid of them.[6] I hate to say this, but sometimes moving to a roach-free living space is the best choice. Short of moving, make sure that there's no food or water left out anywhere in your home. Keep all food sealed in tight containers. Be scrupulously clean. Take the garbage out daily.

Roach baits and boric acid can be helpful in controlling cockroaches, but be careful about roach sprays. The strong chemicals in most roach sprays can be asthma triggers themselves.

Caulking can also help by eliminating all those cracks and crevices that the roaches use to get in and out of your home. Find and fill any holes in the walls. Caulk any openings around pipes or plumbing. And use caulking to seal the cracks in your food cabinets.

As with dust mites and other allergens, an allergy test can tell you how aggressive you need to be.

Mold

Molds and mildew are fungi that liberate spores. Just like the pollen from plants, the tiny mold spores can be inhaled into the lungs. The allergic reaction to the mold spore can trigger runny noses, itchy eyes, and asthma.

Molds can grow both indoors and outdoors. Outdoor mold spore levels tend to peak in the late summer to early fall. Contact the National Allergy Bureau (see appendix C) to find mold spore counts for your area.

Decaying vegetation and compost may be rich with mold spores.[7] Children who are highly mold allergic should avoid raking leaves and cutting grass (or at least wear an allergen-proof mask when doing so).

Indoor molds love warm, humid, and musty places. These are not limited to damp parts of the kitchen, bathroom, laundry room, closets, basement, and other moist or poorly ventilated rooms. If your roof leaks, mold is probably growing in the walls.

Humidifiers are a big source of mold—even when you clean them, the damp air promotes mold growth (dust mites thrive with high humidity also). Humidifier use can make asthma worse. I grew up believing that humidification was good for breathing, and was surprised when I read studies that clearly showed worse asthma control in homes where humidifiers were used.[8]

Humidifiers and vaporizers are almost always a bad idea for people with asthma. However, if you live in a dry climate and feel that some humidification is needed, buy a humidity gauge so that you can keep humidity levels between 30 and 50 percent. Below 30 percent is uncomfortable; dust mites and molds thrive at humidity levels above 50 percent.

Go through your home and look for mold, mildew, and moisture. Look at what may be contributing to it—where is the moisture supporting it coming from? Is there a plumbing leak or roof leak? Is mold accumulating by an overwatered house plant? How about the refrigerator drip pan?

To control mold, decrease humidity and increase ventilation. Sometimes leaving a light on in the closet, or keeping the bathroom window cracked open, can help. In moist areas, a dehumidifier may be necessary.

There are many mold-removal products on the market, however, bleach remains one of the best and cheapest ways to control mold growth.

Pollen and Grasses

If you were a plant, you would think that pollen was sexy. Pollens are the microspores that wind or insects carry from plant to plant so that their seeds may become fertilized. Without pollen, there is no fertilization. Without fertilization, there are no seeds, nuts, grains, or fruit.

On the other hand, if you are a human with asthma, pollen often represents an asthma and allergy trigger. Short of moving, you're pretty much stuck with the pollen in your region.

When pollen counts are high, take extra precautions. Keep windows closed, and consider using air conditioning if needed.

If pollen triggers your child's asthma, more preventive medicine may be needed during the pollen season—and less the rest of the year. Pollen counts tend to be at their highest during the spring and summer. Contact the National Allergy Bureau (see appendix C) to find out about pollen counts in your area.

Allergy testing can tell if pollen can be a problem for your child.

ALLERGY TESTING

Allergy testing can help you tell if an allergen is contributing to your child's asthma.

Skin Tests
The skin-prick test is one of the best ways to find out what you are allergic to. An allergist or an allergy nurse will do the skin testing.

Skin testing can't be done if your child's skin welts when scratched. Asthma must be in good control prior to skin testing. Even a mild asthma flare-up will increase the risk for a severe adverse reaction to a skin test.

Antihistamines (allergy medicine) may block the skin test reaction. Make sure your child doesn't take an antihistamine before skin testing. The effect of some of the newer (prescription) antihistamines can last for weeks to months. Be sure that your allergist knows what medications your child has taken and when the last dose was. Keep in mind that many cough and cold medicines contain antihistamines.

To perform a skin-prick test, a drop of allergen is applied to the skin and a small prick of the skin is made through that drop of allergen. If a large welt develops at the site, your child is likely allergic to that substance.

Though skin-prick testing is good, it isn't perfect. Some people may have negative skin tests but still be allergic. If a substance brings out allergy or asthma symptoms, it is probably best to avoid it—whatever the allergy test results show.

Skin testing can be performed on children of any age—even infants. But keep in mind that even if a child's test is negative, he or she can still develop an allergy later.

Blood Testing

An antibody called immunoglobulin E (IgE) is associated with allergies. A type of blood test called RAST (Radio Allergosorbent Test) testing looks for the specific IgE antibody targeted to an allergen (an allergen is a substance that can trigger an allergic reaction).

The advantage of RAST testing is that it is a simple blood test. The results are not affected by medications. Blood for a RAST test can be drawn no matter how bad the asthma control is.

A strong positive result on a RAST test can be believed—this is evidence of allergy.

The problem with the RAST blood test is that sometimes a child can have a negative result and still be allergic to that allergen. A negative RAST test does not rule out a problem. If an allergen is suspected and the RAST test is negative, often a skin test needs to be done to follow up.

Foods

Though many people with food allergies may have asthma, only a small proportion of children with asthma alone have food allergies.

Here's why: What you inhale goes directly to the lungs. What you eat, however, goes to your whole body. It would be unusual for a food allergy to affect the lungs but not other parts of the body. Usually you'd see things like skin rashes.

Sometimes the food allergy is obvious. If within minutes of eating a peanut your child is coughing, wheezing, and breaking out in welts all over the body, any parent will know what is going on.

However, most of the time the picture is not so simple. The infant drinks milk all the time and wheezes all the time. Is it cause and effect? Maybe. Maybe not.

Diagnosing a food allergy is difficult. The reason is that frequently an allergy test for a food may be positive when the food is not causing any trouble whatsoever. This is what we call a "false positive."

The gold standard for diagnosis of food allergy is the double-blind food challenge. A capsule that might have the food or might have placebo in it is ingested (neither you nor your doctor know which it is). If a reaction is repeatedly produced after the food and not after placebo, you have a clear, definite diagnosis. But doing this is expensive and time-consuming. It is rarely done in clinical practice.

Most of the time the diagnosis of food allergy is based on a combination of allergy testing and an educated guess. If the test is positive and the patient has a history of compatible symptoms, the allergy to the food is likely.

Should we be extra cautious and just eliminate any food that might be a culprit? For children who test positive for many foods this could be a problem. There may be very little left that they can eat. More than a few children inappropriately diagnosed with multiple food allergies have become malnourished.

When should food allergy be suspected? When asthma is combined with other allergic disorders, such as eczema (a scaly, itchy allergic skin rash). Food allergy may be a present in close to one-third of children with moderate to severe eczema.[9] The most commonly implicated foods include milk, egg, peanut, soy, and wheat.

If eczema and asthma coexist, a search for food allergy may pay off. Or, if there is an obvious reaction shortly after eating a food, allergy should be suspected. An allergist can do the appropriate testing to find out.

Non-allergic Triggers

Some substances can trigger asthma, but not via the allergic route. Allergy testing won't help sort the following out.

Aerosol Sprays

Hair sprays, deodorants, room deodorizers—just about anything that comes in a can with a spray nozzle can trigger asthma. It is an irritant—not an allergen. Almost all persons with asthma will benefit from avoiding aerosol sprays.

Find alternatives to sprays. Use a mousse or styling gel for the hair. Change to a roll-on or stick deodorant. Avoid "deodorizers" and "air fresheners."

Keep the air in your home as chemical-free as possible. What you spray in the air will end up in your children's lungs.

Anything with a Strong Smell

Products such as strong-smelling cleansers and solvents can also trigger asthma. Likewise perfumes. Even live Christmas trees are an offender: their pine oil, as well as the pollens and molds they carry, are all asthma triggers. A general rule of thumb: If it smells strong, it may be an asthma trigger.

Aspirin

Aspirin can trigger asthma. Five to 10 percent of adults with moderate to severe asthma may be aspirin sensitive. On the other hand, aspirin-induced asthma is unusual (but not unheard of) in children.

Other aspirinlike drugs such as ibuprofen (Advil, Motrin) can trigger similar reactions. A good alternative is acetaminophen (Tylenol, Tempra, Panadol, etc.), as it does not trigger asthma.

The signs of aspirin sensitivity can be subtle. Typically, the tightening of the breathing tubes starts slowly, about thirty minutes to two hours after taking the aspirin. The reaction resolves slowly.

Correctly diagnosing aspirin-induced asthma may be tough. Was the asthma triggered by the aspirin or by the cold that prompted you to take the aspirin or ibuprofen in the first place?

My own feeling is that if there is any question about aspirin sensitivity, it's probably safest to avoid aspirin and ibuprofen.

Of course, it is best to avoid aspirin in children anyway, because it has been associated with a rare, severe neurologic (brain) disorder called Reye syndrome.

Changes in the Weather

There's not much you can do about the weather, but it's worth knowing that a change in it can trigger an asthma episode. Cold snaps—when the air becomes dry and chilled—are especially likely to trigger asthma.

To keep the breathing tubes from narrowing after exposure to cold, dry air, have your child wear a scarf or mask over the nose and mouth when going outside during the winter. It will help to prewarm and prehumidify the air.

Infections

In years past, much of asthma was misdiagnosed as bronchitis and treated with antibiotics, which in most cases did no good at all.

However, sometimes infections *are* important triggers of asthma. A sinus infection is a common cause of an asthma flare-up that's slow to resolve. The most common symptom of a sinus infection is a green to yellow nasal discharge that won't go away. It's particularly suspicious if the discharge is from one side of the nose only.

Diagnosis of sinus infections can be tricky. I've seen sinus infections diagnosed when they weren't really there, and overlooked when they really were there. (At various times in my career I have been guilty of both.)

Lots of times a parent will come to me the moment that their child's mucus turns green and ask for antibiotics. That's too soon in many cases. Green mucus for two to three days is common as a cold is clearing up. The body is cleaning up the damage caused by the virus. Usually in these cases, however, the child is starting to feel better even though the discharge is green.

On the other hand, if yellow to green pus comes out of the nose for more than seven to ten days, and the chest remains tight, I'm suspicious of a sinus infection—especially if it is accompanied by persistent asthma symptoms.

Though, to be fair, I have to say that many times I have seen sinus infections where the only manifestation was asthma that just wouldn't clear up. If an asthma exacerbation is not improving—or is getting worse—after several days of treatment, see your doctor. An infection might be the reason.

Diagnosing a sinus infection is important because this is one case where treatment with antibiotics will help your asthma. I have had many patients for whom we could not get their asthma under control until the sinus infection was diagnosed and treated.

Preventing Infections

There are simple things you and your child can do to effectively prevent infections. The simplest and most important is for everyone to wash their hands—often. Colds are passed from hand to nose.

Another simple thing is to get a flu shot (influenza vaccine) every year for your children and yourself. Influenza is the one viral trigger of asthma that is preventable. Flu shots for each year usually become available between late September and mid-October. It is important to get the flu shot well before the flu season starts (usually December or January).

Exercise

This can be a scary one for children and parents alike. It's true that exercise can bring on a flare-up, but kids need exercise (adults, too). Exercise is important for the health of the heart and lungs. Asthma shouldn't prevent your child from exercising or playing sports. Because you can anticipate the problem, you can take some simple measures to prevent it.

Vigorous exercise alone can trigger asthma. Sometimes, however, it is the cold, dry air. Or the pollen and/or mold spores in the play area trigger the asthma.

Swimming doesn't provoke asthma nearly as much as other sports, so that's often a good choice. But if asthma is well controlled, your child should be able to participate in any sport he or she wishes.

Sometimes exercise-induced asthma is the only manifestation of asthma. If there is coughing, wheezing, and/or chest tightness right after vigorous exercise, consider that exercise-induced asthma may be present.

Asthma has not prevented elite athletes from achieving excellence. Sixteen percent of the summer 1996 U.S. Olympic team reported a history of asthma or use of asthma medication.[10] Winter Olympic participants had even more, with 22 percent of the 1998 U.S. team having asthma.[11]

Jackie Joyner-Kersee, for example, conquered severe, life-threatening asthma to become one of the world's fastest women, taking the Olympic Gold in 1988 and setting several world records in track and field competition.

Asthma should not hold a kid back from exercise or sports participation. Rather, asthma should be controlled so that that kid—your child—can get out there and conquer the world.

Preventing Exercise-Induced Asthma

With simple precautions, asthma doesn't have to limit participation in sports and exercise. Keeping the underlying asthma well controlled is important; however, medication taken shortly before exercise is key:

- Albuterol (Proventil, Ventolin). One or two puffs given 15 to 30 minutes before exercise works best.
- Cromolyn (Intal) or nedocromil (Tilade). Two puffs before exercise can also be useful (though it is somewhat less effective than albuterol, it also has less side effects).
- Salmeterol (Serevent). Taken in the morning it may help prevent some exercise-induced symptoms during the day. Although it may be more convenient, it is not as effective as albuterol taken just before exercise.

If your child is exercising outdoors in cold, dry air (for example, playing touch football), have him wear a scarf or mask over the face to warm the air as he breathes.

Always have a quick-relief inhaler (such as albuterol) easily available when exercising. Sometimes an exercise-induced asthma attack can be severe. *Not taking proper precautions and not having medication available can be dangerous.*

REAL-WORLD STRATEGIES

Sometimes when we run down our list of asthma triggers with parents, we can see their shoulders slump and their eyes glaze over. It seems like too much to take on.

But I see it in a different light. Each item on this list could represent an *opportunity* to improve your child's health.

You don't have to take on everything at once. Do what you can do now. Focus efforts on the bedroom. Feel good about the excellent start you have made. Go for the simplest measures with the highest-payoff measures first.

Controlling Asthma Triggers: The Big Payoffs
Here are some of the most effective steps you can take to control asthma triggers in your home:

1. **Throw away the ashtrays.**
   Keep the home smoke free.
2. **Make your child's bedroom an allergy-free zone.**
   Control dust mites with allergen-proof encasings on the mattress, box spring, and pillow. Wash all bedding (and stuffed animals) in hot water. Minimize clutter.
3. **Build a dog (or cat) house.**
   Keep pets OUT of the bedroom. If possible, keep them out of the house entirely.
3. **Get rid of the humidifier.**
4. **Keep the air in your home clean.**
   Avoid using aerosol sprays, deodorizers, and strong chemicals inside your home.
5. **Be sure your family gets annual flu shots.**

Controlling Triggers outside the Home

If you follow the steps outlined in this chapter to control asthma triggers in and around your home, you've taken a huge step in the right direction.

As you look at other environments, the most obvious ones are day care, school, and camp, where kids spend most of the rest of their time.

You'll also want to think about friends' and relatives' homes. The most important thing to look for is smoke. If your child spends a lot of time at a friend's house where one or both parents smoke, you could be inviting trouble. In such circumstances, you might insist they play outside, or at your house.

Sleepovers are another potential problem. Bedding is part of the problem, but there's also the issue of your child forgetting to take his or her medication or feeling awkward about taking it. However, with proper management, your child doesn't have to be a social outcast. Send your own bedding if kids are bunking down. Your child can use the inhaler in the bathroom if that feels less conspicuous. Let the host parent know about the asthma. Give them a copy of your child's written asthma management plan (see chapter 9) so they know what to do.

Asthma Triggers in School or Day Care

Occupational asthma is well established in adults—triggered by the variety of chemicals and allergens that many of us may be exposed to at work. For children, going to school is their occupation. Many asthma triggers may be hiding in the school.

There may be furry or feathered pets in the classroom. Poorly maintained schools may have problems with dust, mold, or cockroaches. Arts and crafts or science lab supplies may be used in areas with inadequate ventilation. Grass may be cut during the school day. And don't forget about the potential for passive smoke exposure from other students or from teachers.

Sometimes, just pointing out the problem will motivate the school to do something about it. Other times a note from your doctor may be needed. Occasionally, parents have had to address the problem with the school principal, school superintendent, or school board. Only rarely should it be necessary to pull a child out of a school.

A Word about Pollution

Pollution can be a trigger for asthma. On days with low air quality, you'll want to keep your child indoors as much as possible (which shouldn't be too difficult, since those days tend to be hot and miserable anyway).

Be aware of pollution sources in your neighborhood. It may be an industrial plant or refinery. Or a bus depot or truck stop—burning all that diesel fuel can trigger asthma. Certain agricultural practices such as burning of fields or spraying crops can cause problems in neighboring areas. Control of these pollution sources may take a commitment to political action.

Smog can come not only from large industrial sites but also from sources like automobiles, fireplaces, and charcoal grills. Much as we'd all like to blame other folk for polluting the air, the fact is we all have a hand in it. Though some improvements have been made, more are needed. Improving air quality will take all of us working together.

While political and environmental action are important, I've met some parents who put *too much* emphasis on the effects of pollution—to the point that it makes them feel powerless on a day-to-day level. The reality is that the environment in and around your home is likely to have a far greater impact than air pollution. That's something you *do* have control over, and that's where you can do the most for your child.

7

Managing the Breathing Tubes

Remember the story of Maricella from chapter 2? When I first met her, she was going from crisis to crisis. Her quick-relief inhaler allowed only a brief respite from asthma symptoms. We started a daily medicine to make her breathing tubes less sensitive. The crises became less frequent. She began to feel normal.

The second line of defense against asthma is to make the breathing tubes less sensitive. Then when asthma triggers do get through, they're like a seed landing on rocky ground. They can't get a foothold.

The basic idea is this: It's a lot easier to *prevent* inflammation than to *reverse* it once it gets started. Inflammation acts sort of like a chain letter—when cells receive a chemical signal that says "inflammation," they turn around, amplify the signal and send it out to others. Pretty soon reinforcements have arrived from all over the body, creating more inflammation.

The medications we review in this chapter are all used to keep those first signals from kicking in. Each class of medicine uses a different strategy to block the inflammation. We'll look at how they work and how to keep the side effects at bay. We'll also go over the unique advantages and disadvantages of each of the different medications—so that working with your doctor you can choose the best medicines for your children.

The biggest challenge you'll face with these medications is getting kids to use them consistently.

Kids—and adults, for that matter—would be more likely to take these medications if they felt an immediate improvement in their lungs afterward. But these drugs work slowly. In most cases it takes about two weeks to start to see a measurable improvement, and over a month to get the maximum benefit. We'll explore ways to work taking the medicine into your daily routine.

The Medications

Several classes of drugs can help reduce the breathing tubes' sensitivity. The most potent and easiest to use are the inhaled corticosteroids. A different class of medicines, the chromones, have an excellent safety profile, but they aren't very potent. The "leukotriene modifiers" are the newest class of asthma-preventing medication. I have listed the names of the different medications in each class in the table below.

Medications to Make the Breathing Tubes Less Sensitive

Inhaled Corticosteroids	Chromones	Leukotriene Modifiers

Metered dose inhalers
beclomethasone (Beclovent,
   Vanceril, Vanceril DS, QVAR)
triamcinolone acetonide
   (Azmacort)
flunisolide (AeroBid,
   Aerobid M)
fluticasone (Flovent)
 	
Dry Powder Inhaler
budesonide (Pulmicort)
fluticasone (Flovent Rotadisk)
 	
Nebulizer Machine
budesonide (Pulmicort Respules)
	Nebulizer
	cromolyn (Intal)
	
	Metered Dose Inhaler
	cromolyn
	   (Intal)
	nedocromil
	   (Tilade)
		Pills
		montelukast
		   (Singulair)
		zafirlukast
		   (Accolate)
		zileuton
		   (Zyflo)

Inhaled Corticosteroids

Over the years, the inhaled corticosteroids have proven to be the best preventive medications we have to protect the lungs against asthma. They work at the level of the individual cells, muting almost all of the different chemical signals that lead to inflammation.

Most people tolerate low to moderate doses of an inhaled corticosteroid medicine quite well. Parents tend to like the convenience of having to administer them only a couple of times a day. They also like the effectiveness—how regular use of the medication keeps the asthma under control.

Remember: These medicines, if used every day, *prevent* asthma symptoms from starting. They are very good at keeping the inflammation of the breathing tubes at bay. They are not good at reversing the inflammation that is already there. They do not provide quick relief. They take weeks to work. Once a flare-up is under way we use other medications, which we'll look at in the next chapter.

You can tell whether the inhaled steroids are working, not minute to minute, or day to day—but month to month. Asthma symptoms become less frequent and less severe. Your child's quick-relief inhaler is lasting a lot longer. Measurements of lung function improve. But they don't make symptoms go away if your child is having an asthma flare-up.

This distinction is critical. Parents who believe inhaled steroids are for "treatment of asthma symptoms" are much less likely to use them daily than parents who believe that they "prevent asthma from starting."[1] It really shouldn't be surprising that our beliefs affect our actions.

Safety of Inhaled Steroids

Many parents (and doctors, too) are concerned about the safety of the inhaled corticosteroids. I am often asked, "Aren't they like the steroids I see athletes abusing?" and "Will they hurt my child's liver?" The answer to both is no. The steroids that athletes abuse are called "androgenic steroids," a very different type of drug.

Inhaled corticosteroids are also different from oral corticosteroids. Inhaled medicine does not have to pass through your toes just to get to your lungs. Because you can put a tiny amount of medicine right where you need it, the inhaled steroids can help the lungs without having much effect elsewhere in the body. This is what makes the inhaled steroids so much safer for long-term use.

A lot of careful research has been done looking at side effects of inhaled corticosteroids.[2] When they first became popular, doctors were concerned about three major issues: effects on the bones, effects on the eyes, and effects on growth.

Bones

We know that long-term (months or years) use of oral corticosteroids *can* weaken bones. Low to moderate doses of an *inhaled* corticosteroid *do not*.

I became reassured about the inhaled corticosteroids after I read studies in which sophisticated measures were unable to show any change in bone density among children on low to moderate doses of inhaled steroids.[3]

In fact, if you think about it, these drugs may *help* the bones. Here's why: If asthma isn't well controlled, your child will have more flare-ups. During a flare-up, we often must resort to using oral corticosteroids. So without the flare-ups, there is less need for oral corticosteroids, and hence, less risk of damage to the bones.

Furthermore, if asthma is in good control, your child can be more active. There is nothing like vigorous exercise to build and strengthen bones.

Eyes

We were also concerned about the eyes. Oral corticosteroids, used for long periods of time, can cause cataracts. A large study (published in the *New England Journal of Medicine*) looked at the risk of cataracts associated with use of inhaled corticosteroids. Researchers did find a small increase in the risk of cataracts among older adults who used inhaled steroids.[4] The effect, however, seemed to be dose related—higher doses caused most of the problems.

Fortunately, children seem to have been spared. *Not one cataract in a child has been associated with taking inhaled corticosteroids.*[5] So I am reassured that the risk of cataracts is small, only affects older adults, and can be minimized by using low to moderate doses of inhaled steroids.

Growth

Perhaps the area that has caused the most concern and controversy is the issue of growth. When taken for years at high doses, oral corticosteroids are known to stunt growth. In studies of children who used inhaled corticosteroids, some have found no effect, and others show only a very small slowing of the growth rate. Again, the effect seems to be dose related. It is more prominent at the higher doses, with little if any effect at low doses.

This effect has been difficult to study, because poorly controlled asthma itself can slow growth rates. Further complicating the research is the fact that children don't grow evenly and smoothly, but in spurts. The most important outcome is not what happens to growth over a few months, or even a year or two. The most important outcome is final adult height.

Dr. Søren Pedersen and his colleagues in Denmark have done important work in this area. Their studies found small decreases in short-term (several weeks) growth rate in children taking inhaled steroids.[6] Differences were small and found only at moderate to high doses; no effect was seen with low doses.

One high-quality study compared moderate doses of beclomethasone to placebo (an inactive substance that's used as a control in these types of studies). After the first three months, the group receiving beclomethasone had grown an average of 1 cm (a little less than a half-inch) less than the control group. For the rest of the year, growth rates were similar. Asthma control was much better in the beclomethasone-treated group.[7]

Is this half-inch decrease in growth a one-time event or does each year bring a further decrease? A recently published long-term study is reassuring.

The Childhood Asthma Management Program (CAMP) is a landmark study of childhood asthma. One thousand forty-one children were studied. They were followed for up to six years, which alone makes it a powerful study. Small differences between groups can be detected. They compared children taking budesonide (an inhaled corticosteroid) with children taking nedocromil (a nonsteroidal asthma preventer) or placebo. After six years, the children receiving the inhaled corticosteroid grew only a half-inch less than their peers in the placebo group.[8]

In exchange for this, the children taking the inhaled corticosteroid had much better asthma control. They needed 43 percent less oral steroids (such as prednisone), 45 percent fewer emergency visits, and 43 percent fewer hospitalizations. They had more asthma symptom–free days. And they felt better about themselves.

What about their final adult height? A child's "target" adult height can be estimated from the height of the parents. Drs. Agertoft and Pedersen carefully examined how well children with asthma on inhaled corticosteroid medication reached their target adult height. The reassuring news: By the time they stopped growing, their average height was the same as the average of their target heights. The same was true of their healthy siblings. Final adult height was not affected by their inhaled corticosteroid medication.[9]

My own experience is similar. Most children follow their growth curve at or slightly below where they were before they started the medicine.

How to I make sense out of this? A low to moderate daily dose of an inhaled corticosteroid does have a small effect on growth. The effect on final adult height seems to be minimal. On the other hand, the benefit, in terms of improved asthma control, is large.

LESS IS MORE?

Provocative studies by William Busse, M.D., of the University of Wisconsin (Madison), made many of us question our belief that "if a little is good, more is better." He showed that most of the benefit from inhaled corticosteroids comes at low to moderate doses.[10] At higher doses there are many more side effects but only little benefit.

In other words, most of the benefit from inhaled corticosteroids can be obtained at the lower doses that cause minimal to no side effects.

There are other mild side effects that are occasionally seen with inhaled corticosteroid medications.

Hoarseness

For most patients, this side effect isn't noticeable, especially if a spacer device is used. Dry powder inhalers (such as the Pulmicort Turbuhaler) seem to cause less hoarseness than metered-dose inhalers.

Cough

Some people will cough after using an inhaler. This is usually not a problem. Rarely, the "inactive" ingredients in a metered-dose inhaler can cause enough irritation to the throat to create a chronic cough.

It can sometimes be difficult to decide if the cough is due to asthma, due to the asthma inhaler, or due to something else. If lung function is normal, the quick-relief inhaler doesn't help control the cough, and no other cause for the cough can be found, discuss with your doctor the possibility that the asthma inhaler might be causing the cough.

Thrush

Thrush is a yeast infection in the mouth. It's easy to detect, since you can see white spots on the inside of the cheeks. They look a little like milk, but you can't rinse them away. Thrush is caused by the medicine depositing in the mouth. Using a spacer device with the inhaler and rinsing the mouth after the puffs will prevent this problem.

Thrush is easily treated, usually with a safe prescription medicine called Nystatin.

Reducing Side Effects

There are four basic principles to minimizing side effects of inhaled medications:

1. Get it where you need it.

Get more of the medicine into the lungs and less in the mouth and throat. Use a spacer device (such as an AeroChamber or InspirEase) with the metered-dose inhaler (see chapter 12). A good spacer can increase the effective dose (the part that gets to the lungs) while decreasing the total dose (the part that gets to the rest of the body).

Also, have your child rinse and spit after using the inhaler. Medicine on the tongue and cheeks won't help the lungs. It only adds to the side effects. This is probably about the only time that a doctor will say it's OK to spit medicine out.

2. Find the Lowest Effective Dose

Use the lowest dose that will keep asthma in control. Often it's possible to reduce the amount of medications after we get asthma under control. Usually we start inhaled steroid medicines during a time of crisis, so we use a higher dose of medicine to get the asthma quickly into control. Once asthma triggers in the home are controlled and the crisis subsides, say, in a month or two, your child may not need as high a dose to keep the asthma in control.

Remember, though, we're talking here about decreasing the daily dose, not stopping it entirely. Stopping the medicine completely means your child loses the protection against asthma. When the asthma starts acting up again it may take higher doses of medicine to get it back into control. Your child could end up needing *more* medicine.

Follow up with your doctor regularly to make sure that your child's asthma plan is optimal, and to find the lowest medication dose that works. If a daily inhaled steroid medication is needed, your child should see his or her personal physician at least twice a year.[11]

And, of course, be sure to discuss all changes in medications with your doctor.

3. Find the Barriers

If moderate to high doses of inhaled steroids don't control asthma, look for and eliminate the other barriers to good control.

The three most common barriers to good asthma control are (1) poor inhaler technique; (2) not using preventive (inhaled corticosteroid) medicine regularly; and (3) living with an asthma trigger.

Sometimes a complicating medical condition may block asthma control. These include conditions such as sinus infections and gastroesophageal reflux. Gastroesophageal reflux is when acid refluxes out of the stomach into the esophagus (the tube that connects the mouth to the stomach). Sometimes the stomach acid refluxes so high that it can be tasted in the back of the throat. If you think your child may have either of these conditions, talk to your doctor.

Keep in mind that sometimes what we think is asthma may really be something else. If asthma is not controlled despite your best attempts, talk to your doctor. A referral to a pediatric pulmonary or allergy specialist may be needed.

4. Add a "Steroid-Sparing" Medication

If a moderate dose of an inhaled steroid medication does not completely do the job, it may be time to add another medication. Most all of the benefit has already been extracted from this one. Medications that have been shown to have significant benefit when added to a moderate inhaled steroid dose include salmeterol (Serevent), the leukotriene modifiers (Singulair, Accolate), and theophylline (SloBid, TheoDur, Uniphyl, and others). The sections below provide a more in-depth description of these medications.

Comparing the Risks

Sometimes we get so preoccupied with side effects of a medicine that we forget about the side effects of the disease that we are using the medicine to treat.

Poorly controlled asthma can interrupt sleep—so children can't pay attention as well in school. Frequent asthma flare-ups may cause so many school absences that grades suffer.

Poor lung function can keep a child from running and playing—leading to a sedentary lifestyle and increasing the risk of heart disease (the number-one killer of adults in this country) in later life.

New research suggests that years of low-grade inflammation of the breathing tubes can cause permanent damage. The longer you wait to get asthma into control, the worse the lung function and the more severe the asthma.[12] Getting asthma into good control early leads to better long-term outcomes.

And let's not forget the small but significant risk of death from poorly controlled asthma. A recent study shows that even a low dose of inhaled steroid medication taken regularly will decrease the risk of death from asthma.[13]

Choosing an Inhaled Corticosteroid

There are many different inhaled corticosteroid preparations on the market. How do you find the one that is best? The different preparations have their own advantages and disadvantages. My view of the pros and cons of each of them follows, to help you find the preparation that bests suits your needs. You should always talk with your doctor before starting or changing medications.

Beclomethasone (Beclovent, Vanceril, Vanceril DS, QVAR)

What this drug is: Beclomethasone was one of the first inhaled corticosteroids on the market.

Beclovent and Vanceril are metered-dose inhalers with 42 micrograms (that is, 0.042 milligrams) per puff, 200 puffs per canister.

Vanceril DS is a metered-dose inhaler with twice the amount of medicine per puff (84 micrograms = 0.084 milligrams). There are 120 puffs in a Vanceril DS canister.

QVAR is a new formulation of beclomethasone. Its benefit is that it is able to get much more of the medicine dose into the extra-fine particle range—thus more of the dose is able to get deep into the lungs. QVAR does not use chlorofluorocarbons (CFCs) to power the inhaler. The propellant is a substance called hydrofluoroalkane (HFA).

What I like about it: As relatively low-dose preparations, Beclovent and Vanceril are well suited for children with mild persistent asthma. QVAR, if it works the way developers expect, will get more the medicine where it is needed, so a lower dose can be used.

What I don't like about it: If a moderate to high dose of inhaled corticosteroids is needed, lots of puffs of Beclovent or Vanceril may have to be used.

Triamcinolone Acetonide (Azmacort)

What this drug is: Azmacort is an inhaled corticosteroid metered-dose inhaler that comes with a built-in spacer. It delivers 100 micrograms (= 0.10 milligram) per puff, and 240 puffs per inhaler unit.

What I like about it: The built-in spacer is convenient. You don't have to keep track of an "add-on" spacer that is separate from your medicine inhaler.

With 240 puffs in the canister, Azmacort is often one of the more economical choices.

What I don't like about it: Azmacort is not suitable for infants and toddlers who need a spacer with mask (such as the AeroChamber with mask). (See chapter 14 for a full discussion of asthma medication delivery to infants and toddlers.)

Fluticasone (Flovent)

What this drug is: Flovent is a high-potency inhaled corticosteroid metered-dose inhaler. It comes in three strengths (44 micrograms per puff, 110 micrograms per puff, and 220 micrograms per puff), with 120 puffs of medication in each inhaler canister. Flovent is also marketed as a dry powder inhaler in three strengths (50 micrograms, 100 micrograms, and 250 micrograms per dose).

What I like about it: The range of strengths makes it easier to find the right dose while using very few puffs. Side effects are decreased slightly because the liver rapidly inactivates the swallowed part of the dose.

I have had many patients do well with only one or two puffs of this medication daily. You should never need more than two puffs twice daily of Flovent.

What I don't like about it: These formulations make it easy to get to very high doses of this medication with only a few puffs.

As a rule of thumb, for a child I try not to exceed a dose of 440 micrograms per day (2 puffs of the Flovent 220, 4 puffs of Flovent 110). For a teenager or adult, I do not like to use more than 660 micrograms per day (3 puffs of the Flovent 220, 6 puffs of Flovent 110).[14]

Some of my patients complain about the taste of Flovent; others don't seem to mind.

Flunisolide (AeroBid, AeroBid-M)

What this drug is: AeroBid is an inhaled corticosteroid metered-dose inhaler with 250 micrograms per puff, and only 100 puffs per inhaler canister. AeroBid-M is a mint-flavored formulation of the product.

What I like about it: I find nothing special about this product that gives it an advantage over the other inhaled corticosteroids on the market.

What I don't like about it: Many children find the taste of this medicine offensive. Because of the taste, I find it difficult to get kids to take this medicine.

Milligram for milligram, flunisolide is less potent than the other inhaled corticosteroid preparations on the market.

Budesonide Dry Powder Inhaler (Pulmicort Turbuhaler)

What this drug is: Budesonide is an inhaled corticosteroid medication that has been around for a long time in Europe and has only recently been licensed in the United States. The main difference with this product is that it comes as a dry powder inhaler. A dry powder inhaler is a small, compact device. It does not contain a propellant to force the drug out into a spray—all the force comes from your breath. No spacer is needed. The Pulmicort dry powder inhaler delivers 200 micrograms of budesonide per puff, with 200 doses in each canister.

What I like about it: The preparation contains just the pure drug—there are no "inactive" ingredients. It also doesn't have the ozone-layer-damaging chlorofluorocarbons (CFCs) found in other inhalers.

Pulmicort has minimal to no taste. For most people that is a good thing. However, a couple of my patients found the lack of taste disorienting. The taste let them know the medicine was there.

Problems with hoarseness seem to be less frequent with this product.

There's an indicator on the side of the inhaler to let you know when it is running out. This is helpful. Traditional metered-dose inhalers have no such indicator (and may keep spraying even after most of the drug has been emptied from the canister).

What I don't like about it: The Pulmicort dry powder inhaler isn't suitable for young children. A child needs to be old enough to take a deep, rapid forceful breath—typically, about eight years of age or older.

Budesonide for Nebulizer (Pulmicort Respules)

What this drug is: Budesonide is an inhaled corticosteroid medication, used with a nebulizer (a machine that takes liquid medication and makes it into a mist). The mist is inhaled over 7 to 15 minutes through a face mask or mouthpiece.

Budesonide solution for nebulizer has been available for the past decade outside of the United States but has only recently been approved for U.S. markets. It will be marketed in 250 micrograms and 500 micrograms unit dose vials.

What I like about it: Sometimes a nebulizer is easier to give to a young child than a metered-dose inhaler. The mask just needs to be placed on the face. You don't need to make a seal.

What I don't like about it: Medication dosing from a nebulizer is notoriously inefficient. Perhaps 1 percent of the medication dose put into the machine actually makes it into the lungs.

Because some of the mist goes into the air surrounding the child, others in the vicinity may be exposed to low doses of the medication.

Eyes are very sensitive to the effects of corticosteroids. If some of the mist gets into the eyes, risk for cataracts may be increased.

An inhaled corticosteroid given via an AeroChamber with Mask is a perfectly good alternative.

What Inhaled Steroids Should You Avoid?

Some physicians have advised using a nebulizer with corticosteroid preparations that were designed for other uses—such as for the nose (to control allergies) or for injection into a vein (intravenous).[15] Frankly, I can't see any reason to do so. *Stay away from this "off label" use.*

For the nasal corticosteroids (Beconase AQ, Flonase, Nasalide, Rhinocort, etc.), the "inactive" ingredients that are fine for the nose may not be fine for the lungs. The physical properties of the medicine (such as its thickness) may not allow the nebulizer to create small-enough particles to reach deep into the lungs—where the asthma is.

There's nothing to gain by using corticosteroids designed for *intravenous* (IV) use (SoluMedrol, Decadron) in a nebulizer. The corticosteroids designed for inhalation work well locally (in the lungs), but have minimal activity elsewhere. Those designed for IV use, by contrast, work throughout the body. Inhalation of these medicines is just another rapid route to the bloodstream. The margin of safety is lost and the risk for side effects is higher.

Chromones

The chromones include cromolyn (Intal) and nedocromil (Tilade). This class of medication can help block the inflammation that causes asthma, yet they're not corticosteroids.

Cromolyn and nedocromil were developed as synthetic versions of khellin, an herb that has been used medicinally in the Middle East for centuries. Though it is effective for asthma, the pure form of the herb has many troublesome side effects.

The challenge was to develop synthetic forms of khellin that were both effective and safe. Robert Altounyen, a physician of Middle Eastern ancestry, devoted most of his life to this quest. What he came up with were cromolyn and nedocromil. Cromolyn has been around since the 1970s; nedocromil was first licensed in the United States in 1993.

Like the inhaled corticosteroids, cromolyn and nedocromil are long-term controllers of asthma and work by preventing the inflammation that causes asthma. They need to be used every day to prevent asthma from starting; they do not reverse what is already there. They do not provide quick relief of asthma symptoms.

The big problem with the chromones is their lack of potency. You need to use them at least 3–4 times a day each and every day to get the maximum benefit. This can be a big nuisance. A very low dose of an inhaled steroid can help as much or more, and you only have to use it 1–2 times a day.

Chromones work best with mild asthma. I recommend them for patients with mild persistent asthma who want to avoid the inhaled corticosteroids. Chromones tend to be too weak to provide much benefit in moderate to severe asthma.

Safety

The big advantage of the chromone medication is safety. They have zero potential for corticosteroid-like side effects. The most significant side effect I've seen with this class of medications is an occasional cough after using the inhaler. Rare allergic reactions to these medications have been reported. There is no effect on growth, mood, or heart rate.

Cromolyn (Intal)

What this drug is: Cromolyn is a nonsteroid inhaled anti-inflammatory medication. In the United States it is marketed as a metered-dose inhaler delivering 0.80 milligram per puff (200 puffs per canister) and as a solution for nebulization, with 20 milligrams per unit dose.

What I like about it: Excellent track record of safety. Not a steroid.

What I don't like about it: Low potency. You need to use multiple daily doses. It doesn't provide any benefit when added to an inhaled corticosteroid (it's a little like adding a fly swatter to a hammer).

Nedocromil (Tilade)

What this drug is: Nedocromil is a nonsteroid inhaled anti-inflammatory medicine. It is available as a metered-dose inhaler delivering 1.75 mg per puff (112 puffs per canister).

What I like about it: Excellent track record of safety. It may be just a little bit more potent than cromolyn. For a few people, using this medication may allow them to reduce their inhaled corticosteroid dose; however, this benefit tends to be small and inconsistent.

What I don't like about it: About one out of eight people will find the taste of this medication offensive. The rest will find the taste very mild. Like cromolyn, it has a relatively low potency compared to the inhaled steroids.

Leukotriene Modifier Medications

In 1996, the Food and Drug Administration approved the first of a new class of anti-asthma drugs. Like the corticosteroids, they help block inflammation of the breathing passages, and are used to prevent asthma attacks. However, unlike corticosteroids, they only block one part of the inflammatory process—a part called the "leukotriene pathway."

Leukotrienes are a type of chemical messenger that can start up inflammation. Minute quantities released in the lungs can cause a severe asthma attack. You can think of inflammation as a chain of events, sort of like a message transmitted down a battlefield. When an intruder (for example, smoke) is identified on the front lines, the troops send a message back to headquarters to call in the big guns.

Like a message on a battlefield, this message may travel by a variety of routes before it gets to the end of the line. Leukotrienes are one type of "messenger" that can set off the chain reaction.

In asthma, of course, many of these messages are overreactions. These medications use one of two strategies to block the effect of leukotrienes. One type, zileuton (Zyflo), blocks the formation of the leukotrienes.

The other type are the leukotriene receptor antagonists. These medications keep other cells from responding to leukotrienes, thereby effectively blocking their effect. The leukotriene receptor antagonists currently on the market in the United States are zafirlukast (Accolate), and montelukast (Singulair).

When used alone, these medicines work best for mild asthma. Leukotriene modifiers, when used as an add-on drug, may help individuals whose asthma is not completely controlled with a daily inhaled corticosteroid.

Effectiveness varies; for some people, leukotrienes seem to make a major difference. For others, they may not be of much help at all.

Overall, the problem with this class of medication is that there are many other "mediators of inflammation" out there besides leukotrienes. They're just one piece of the puzzle—for some individuals it is the critical piece, for others it is not.

In addition to their preventive qualities, these medications provide some symptom relief. But don't rely on them for that; bronchodilator inhalers like albuterol (see chapter 8) are much more effective.

One advantage of this class of medications is that for people with mild, persistent asthma, there is a pill that can control asthma.

Safety

The leukotriene synthesis inhibitor zileuton (Zyflo) can cause low-grade injury to liver cells in about 2 percent of patients taking it. For this reason, I don't recommend this medicine.

The leukotriene receptor blockers—montelukast (Singulair) and zafirlukast (Accolate)—have an excellent track record of safety so far. They don't seem to cause problems with the liver. The major problem, as I see it, is that this type of medicine is still new. We don't know what long-term effects they may have.

You need to be cautious about the potential for drug interactions, especially with zileuton (Zyflo) and zafirlukast (Accolate). Always check with your doctor or pharmacist to make sure that these drugs are compatible with other medications you may be using.

I prefer the low-dose inhaled corticosteroids to control mild to moderate asthma. We have many years of experience with them, know what the problems are, know how to look for them, and know strategies to reduce the side effects. But if your child has problems with inhaled corticosteroids, the leukotriene receptor blockers are a reasonable second choice.

Zileuton (Zyflo)

What this drug is: A leukotriene synthesis inhibitor. It comes as a pill that is taken four times a day. It is not approved for use in children twelve years and under. Due to its effect on liver function, blood tests to monitor liver enzymes need to be obtained regularly when on this medication.

What I don't like about it: This medication has the potential for low-grade liver injury. The need for up to four-times-a-day dosing is inconvenient. I see no reason to accept these risks and inconveniences when there are good alternatives.

Zafirlukast (Accolate)

What this drug is: A leukotriene receptor blocker. It comes as a pill that is taken twice daily. It is not approved for use in children under seven years of age.

What I like about it: It's a pill that may block mild asthma. In some people (not all) it can provide benefit when combined with an inhaled corticosteroid.

So far, safety seems to be good. Severe problems are rare.

What I don't like about it: It's expensive. It needs to be taken twice a day, and it needs to be taken with food (or the body won't absorb the medicine as well).

It can interact with certain medications (like the blood-thinning medicine warfarin).

Long-term (twenty-plus years) safety is not known.

Montelukast (Singulair)

What this drug is: Leukotriene receptor blocker. It comes as a pill that is taken once daily. It is approved for use in children two years of age and older.

What I like about it: It is a pill that may block mild asthma. It needs to be taken only once a day. It is approved for use in children as young as two years old, and it's available as a chewable tablet, which for many children is easier to take. In some people (not all), it can provide benefit when combined with an inhaled corticosteroid.

So far, safety seems to be excellent.

What I don't like about it: It's expensive. Long-term (twenty-plus years) safety isn't known.

Children using this medication need to learn to take a pill. A liquid formulation is not available.

Long-Acting Symptom Relievers

Sometimes, despite our best efforts, a moderate daily dose of an inhaled corticosteroid doesn't fully control asthma. This is especially true for people with moderate to severe persistent asthma (see chapter 9 for asthma classification). In these cases, adding on a long-acting symptom-relieving medicine is more effective in controlling asthma than going to high-dose inhaled corticosteroids.[16]

The long-acting symptom relievers currently available in the United States include salmeterol (Serevent) and theophylline (SloBid, TheoDur, Uniphyl, etc.).

Salmeterol (Serevent)

What this drug is: Salmeterol (Serevent) is a long-acting symptom reliever for daily use. It is a slow-acting bronchodilator—meaning it works by relaxing the muscle surrounding the breathing tube. It is most effective when used in combination with an inhaled corticosteroid medication. It should *never* be used for quick relief of asthma exacerbations. Never take more than the recommended dose. It takes about half an hour to start working, and lasts for about twelve hours.

Salmeterol comes as a metered-dose inhaler and as a dry powder inhaler. It's not approved for use in children younger than twelve years. A combination of salmeterol with the inhaled corticosteroid fluticasone has just been released as a dry powder inhaler under the brand name of Advair.

What I like about it: If asthma is not completely controlled on a moderate dose of inhaled corticosteroid medication, addition of this medication can improve asthma control. In fact, research has shown that the combination of a moderate dose inhaled steroid with salmeterol gives *better* asthma control than doubling the dose of the inhaled steroid.[17]

What I don't like about it: Though generally this is a good "add-on" medication, it has a few downsides.

It is not approved for use in children under twelve years of age.

It can be stimulating and make the heart beat faster (an effect similar to other bronchodilator medications).

The ability of this medication to block responses to asthma triggers may decrease with chronic use.[18]

Used alone, it is not good anti-asthma therapy. It is most effective when used in combination with an inhaled corticosteroid.

Theophylline (SloBid, TheoDur, Uniphyl, etc.)

Theophylline is in the same class of chemicals as caffeine. It was our mainstay of asthma therapy before the inhaled steroids became popular. The combination of theophylline with a moderate dose of inhaled corticosteroid has been shown to give better asthma control than going to high dose inhaled corticosteroids.[19]

What this drug is: Theophylline is a long-acting bronchodilator (long-acting symptom reliever). Its mechanism of anti-asthma action, though not entirely known, is different from that of albuterol, salmeterol, and other commonly used bronchodilators.

Theophylline is taken orally. It comes in a variety of formulations, from a short-acting liquid to an extended-release tablet or capsule. For young children, the contents of an extended-release capsule can be opened and sprinkled on applesauce or similar acidic food.

What I like about it: Theophylline can improve asthma control when used in combination with an inhaled corticosteroid.

Some people find a medication that can be taken by mouth to be more convenient than an inhaler.

Extended-release preparations are available and effective. Your child needs to take them only once (Uniphyl, others) or twice (SloBid, Theo-Dur, others) a day.

Theophylline is an old and well-characterized medication. We know what trouble we can get into with it and know how to monitor for it.

What I don't like about it: Some children will develop caffeinelike side effects on this medicine, seeming a bit overstimulated. This can be a particular problem for children who are already hyperactive.

An overdose of theophylline can be dangerous, even fatal. Keep the medicine in a safe, secure place. The bioavailability (the amount of medicine taken that gets into the bloodstream) of different brands of theophylline can differ. Consult your doctor before changing brands of theophylline.

Theophylline can have dangerous interactions with other medications, such as erythromycin (an antibiotic) and cimetidine (Tagamet, an antacid), so be sure to check with your doctor or pharmacist to make sure that it is compatible with your child's other medicines.

Like caffeine, theophylline can stimulate gastroesophageal reflux (where acid comes up out of the stomach into the esophagus—food pipe—and sometimes the throat). Gastroesophageal reflux sometimes can trigger asthma.

Allergy Shots: Do They Help?

Allergy shots involve injecting a small amount of an allergen in an attempt to get your body to be tolerant of it.

Allergy shots can give dramatic benefit for people with an allergic runny nose. However, the benefit is often not as dramatic in asthma.

Furthermore, the risk of adverse effects of allergy shots is increased for people with asthma. Keep in mind, we are injecting a small amount of something that, if inhaled, would stimulate coughing and wheezing. Due to the higher risk of adverse reactions, such as stimulating an asthma attack or anaphylactic shock, people with severe or unstable asthma probably should not get allergy shots.

Given these reservations, allergy shots can be helpful in carefully selected people with asthma.[20] Allergy shots are not a first-line treatment. They are not a replacement for asthma medication or environmental control. However, if your child's asthma is not controlled on moderate doses of asthma medication, *and* identifiable allergens are among your child's major triggers, then allergy shots can be of benefit.

Though it is unlikely that allergy shots will allow a child to totally discontinue asthma medication, they can help maintain good asthma control at a lower medication dose.

Allergy shots are best prescribed by an allergist. A series of allergy shots usually starts with a small amount of a low concentration of the allergen extract given one to two times a week. The dose is gradually increased to "maintenance" levels, and the dose interval is lengthened to one to two times per month. It may take from three months to one year to see a benefit from treatment.

To guard against a reaction, it's important that you and your child wait in the doctor's office for at least half an hour after the allergy shot. The clinic must be equipped with trained personnel, medications, and equipment for resuscitation, should there be an adverse reaction to the shot. If there is any evidence of asthma flaring up, the allergy shot should be withheld.[21]

What about Over-the-Counter Cold Medications?

It would be reasonable to assume that over-the-counter medication for colds, allergy symptoms, and sinus problems would help prevent asthma attacks. Unfortunately, that doesn't seem to be the case.

However, I see no reason to suffer with a runny nose when you have asthma. There is no reason that an antihistamine or decongestant can't be used *along with* your asthma medication.

Be cautious about over-the-counter nose spray decongestants such as Neo-Synephrine (active ingredient, phenylephrine). Although it may help for the first couple of days, after a few days of use a "rebound" can occur. After the medicine wears off, the membranes of the nose may swell up. This swelling may be more than your child had before the medicine was used. The increase in swelling after the medicine wears off I call rebound. To minimize the risk of rebound, use of nasal spray (topical) decongestants should be limited to 48 to 72 hours at most.

My pet peeve, however, is cough suppressants. I have seen asthma mistreated with cough medicine more times than I care to recall. A good strong cough is one of the best defenses the lung has. The American Academy of Pediatrics has published a statement advising against the use of cough suppressants in children.[22] For cough, I believe that the best approach is to treat the cause—not just mask the symptom.

Getting Kids to Take Their Medications

The big challenge with using preventive medications is getting kids (adults, too) to use them consistently.

Here's the problem: Instead of making us feel better right away, preventive medications are designed to keep things normal and healthy. When asthma triggers enter the lungs, well, that's about it—you feel just about the same.

It is easy to take medicine when we feel bad. One of the most difficult things to do is to take medicine when we feel well.

For children, other factors may play a role. Younger children may view the inhaler—which is held over the face—as strange and threatening. Older children may view it as a chore—something parents or others make him do. Sometimes taking medicine becomes a power struggle between parent and child. Here are approaches we've found helpful:

Explain why the medicine must be taken

Do this in language that your child can understand. For example, you could explain that the preventive medicines "help your lungs stay normal," "keep asthma away," or "keep your lungs in good shape." For quick-relief medicine, you might say, "This will help you feel better." If the inhaler is blue in color (the popular quick reliever, Ventolin, is blue) you might say, "The blue medicine is for when you feel blue."

Encourage your child to ask questions. I'm often surprised by how readily even very young children catch on. Sometimes drawing pictures or playing games helps them to grasp the concepts.

Set clear and consistent expectations

When it comes to getting out of things they don't want to do, kids are eternal optimists. If they think there's even a chance that you'll let them slide, they'll continue to test you. On the other hand, when parents take a matter-of-fact approach that they must take their medication every day, no ifs, ands, or buts, most kids accept it and it soon ceases to be an issue.

If you want, blame the doctor. Explain that these are doctor's orders, and you really have no choice in the matter.

Provide lots of positive reinforcement

It's human nature to correct a child when they do something wrong more readily than to praise them when they do something right. But positive reinforcement is one of the most powerful—and most underused— tools we have for changing behavior. Notice when things are done well. Give rewards for the desired behaviors. Praise is often the best motivation. Often a star chart is helpful—when they take their medicine well, they get a gold star. The gold stars are negotiable. Three stars, for example, might earn a small prize or privilege, such as getting to watch a favorite TV program. Twenty stars might be exchanged for a more valuable item. Agree with your child on the rules beforehand and write them down. Be definite about exactly what behaviors earn gold stars as well as exactly what the gold stars will buy.

Prioritize

Don't target too many things for change right away. Start with the one or two most important changes. It makes me cringe when I hear a parent tell the child to "be sure to take your medicine, and clean your room, and do the dishes, eat your vegetables, clean your fingernails . . ."

and so on. (Of course, the same could be said for doctors who give families a huge laundry list of changes to make.)

Build routines

I often find that if I have to "remember" to do something each day, it may get done—or it may not. Taking medicine tends to fall to the low end of the priority list. But if it's linked to something that we already do as a routine, it's more likely to get done.

In my experience, one of the best routines to attach to is brushing the teeth. Keep the inhaler in the bathroom. Have your child use it first, then brush his teeth. That gets three birds with one stone: It builds on a habit they already have. It helps kill the taste, which some kids find objectionable. Perhaps most important, it ensures that they'll wash out their mouths after using the inhaler.

You can use other routines, too: getting dressed or undressed, before breakfast or dinner—whatever seems to work best. Sometimes it helps to have reminders in key locations. Place a note on the bathroom mirror, the dresser, or the bedroom door. For me, it helps to have the note on the door I leave the house from. Or you may want to check off on a calendar whether your child took the medicine.

As your child starts to demonstrate maturity in taking medication, you can give her more responsibility. That may mean, for example, trusting her to take her medication without you standing over her. Ultimately, the goal is to transfer responsibility to the child, so that later on in life these habits will be second nature.

You can still check that the asthma prevention medicines are being taken because: (1) their asthma stays well controlled; (2) the long-term inhalers become empty after an appropriate time (see table below; and (3) quick-relief medicines (like albuterol) are needed infrequently.

Rewards don't only have to be things like treats or presents. They can be anything that makes the behavior more likely. For example, as your child continues to use the preventive medications, you can help him or her look for the differences. Your child won't notice them day to day. But after a couple of weeks, he may find that he's coughing and wheezing less often and the quick-relief inhalers are lasting longer. If she monitors her lung function with a peak flow meter, she'll find that her best is getting better and that there are fewer dips. Give praise as you notice how well controlled the asthma is.

How Long Will an Inhaler Last?

	# puffs (per canister)	1 puff/day	2 puffs/day	4 puffs/day	6 puffs/day	8 puffs/day
AeroBid	100	n/a	50 days	25 days	16 days	12 days
Serevent	120	n/a	60 days	30 days	n/a	n/a
Flovent	120	120 days	60 days	30 days	20 days	15 days
Beclovent Vanceril	200	n/a	100 days	50 days	33 days	25 days
Pulmicort	200	200 days	100 days	50 days	33 days	25 days
Azmacort	240	n/a	120 days	60 days	40 days	30 days

On the inhaler, mark the date when you start using it. Using the table above, based on the dose taken, determine how long the inhaler should last. Then mark the date that you *expect* the inhaler to be empty. Make sure the medicine is refilled at least 1 week before your supply runs out. Don't be caught empty.

We have found that it's useful to keep a written record to track these improvements. It creates a visible measure of improvement that helps keep motivation high, and it's great for communication with your doctor as well.

8

Managing Flare-Ups

When I first met Jeremy, he wanted to live his life and ignore his asthma. His parents smoked, but they tried to keep it outside the house. He had frequent bouts of coughing and wheezing. When they got so bad he couldn't stand it, he would take a couple of puffs on his quick-relief inhaler. He tried to ignore his asthma.

The second time I met him, he was on a ventilator in the emergency room.

He'd been out playing basketball, developed an asthma attack, used his inhaler, and went home. His dad took one look at him and brought him into the emergency room. He barely made it. Dad burst through the doors and dropped Jeremy onto a gurney. It took only a couple of seconds for the doctors to realize that Jeremy had stopped breathing. They quickly had him intubated and put on the ventilator. They called me to come down to help get him stabilized. Before his parents left, I told them that by working together we could prevent this from ever happening again.

After leaving the hospital, Karen—one of our asthma nurse case managers—and I contacted the family. Working together with Jeremy and his family, we developed an asthma management program. After nearly losing Jeremy, they didn't have any hesitation in following it. He and his parents learned what to do to keep minor problems from escalating.

Now Jeremy is one of our "poster children" for good asthma management. He is back playing basketball. He's doing well in high school. He's very popular with the girls in his school. And he hasn't been back to the emergency room.

. . .

When parents, doctors, and children are aggressive about the first two lines of defense—managing the environment and managing the breathing tubes—flare-ups tend to be a lot less frequent. They're usually milder, more easily controlled—and a lot less frightening.

The third line of defense is to create an early-warning system so that we can see flare-ups coming and take *early* action.

As parents and kids learn more about their asthma and become better attuned to it, they can tell when problems are brewing. They learn what's likely to set off a flare-up. And they learn how to listen to their lungs.

We follow three basic principles for managing asthma flare-ups:

1. We work to prevent them by controlling asthma triggers and, if needed, by using preventive medicines. If a patient is having asthma flare-ups, it suggests that we need to reexamine our first two lines of defense—managing the environment and managing the breathing tubes.

2. We help kids and their parents recognize the flare-up early. An asthma flare-up is like a fire burning in the lungs. Early detection makes it easier to control.

3. We recognize and take prompt action to reverse the flare-up, before it gets out of control.

The Peak Flow Meter:
Your Early-Warning System

One of the biggest problems we face in managing flare-ups is waiting too long to get started. The reasons are understandable. Good, concerned parents don't want to overreact and subject their children to medications they don't need. They're inclined to wait and see before they hit the panic button. But it's a lot easier to manage a flare-up that's four hours old than to manage one that's forty-eight hours old.

Some parents tell me they don't want to "bother" the doctor until they're sure. Trust me: It's no bother. I'd much rather see a child in the early stages of a flare-up during regular office hours than to see him or her in crisis at 2 A.M. in the emergency room.

You can use two strategies for early detection. One is monitoring asthma symptoms. A much better strategy is to monitor your peak flow.

The peak flow meter is a simple, inexpensive device that measures lung function. You can use it to find out how open or closed the breathing tubes are. Most children over five or six years of age are able to use it.

The peak flow meter is a device that measures how hard a person can breathe out. The greater the force they use when they blow into the meter, the higher the peak flow reading (the technical term is peak expiratory flow rate). So, in other words, high scores are good.

To use a peak flow meter, have your child fill his lungs completely then blow into the meter with all his might. When your child's breathing tubes are tightening, he won't be able to blow out with as much force as when the breathing tubes are fully open. In an asthma flare-up, a diminished peak flow is usually the first sign to appear. As a result, the peak flow meter helps you spot an asthma flare-up in its earliest stages.

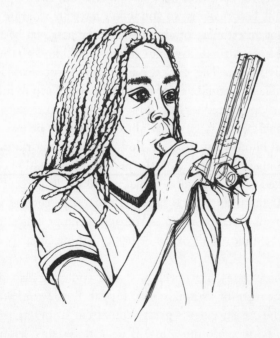

Using a peak flow meter to measure lung function

The peak flow meter is also a more reliable measure of severity of a flare-up than symptoms are. Lung function starts to decline well before there's any noticeable difference in breathing. That's especially true with kids. Their lungs have lots of excess capacity, so they—and you—may not notice anything wrong at first.

Most people need to lose about a quarter of their lung function before they notice a difference (some a little more, others a bit less). Studies show that those with the *most severe* asthma are the *least sensitive* to difficulties in breathing, presumably because they've lived with diminished lung capacity for so long it feels normal.[1]

Anne, for example, had a history of severe asthma. On one of her first visits to me, she told me she felt okay. When I listened to her chest, her breath sounds were normal. Yet when I checked her peak flow rate, it was very low. I confirmed that with a full set of lung function tests, and found that her breathing tubes were severely tightened.

To find out how tight your child's breathing tubes are, compare the current peak flow to his or her "personal best" peak flow.

You find your child's personal best peak flow when asthma is in good control. If you only check the peak flow when your child is ill, you won't know what the best really is, so you won't have an accurate measure.

If you want an estimate of about where the personal best should be, look at a table of normal (average) values (you'll find a table in appendix B of this book). The package insert for most peak flow meters includes a table of normal values for their meter. Keep in mind that the "normal" or "predicted" peak flow is just an average value. Your child's personal best may be either above average or below.

The actual number on the peak flow isn't too important. The key is how that number compares with the personal best. Asthma is generally well controlled if the peak flow is within 80 or 90 percent of the personal best. If the peak flow is below 50 or 60 percent of your child's best, it means a severe flare-up is starting. Prompt action needs to be taken, because almost half of his or her breathing capacity has already been lost.

If peak flow rates are checked daily, you will also get another important measure of asthma control: peak flow *variability*. In other words, are the measurements pretty consistent from day to day, or do they tend to bounce around a lot? If peak flows stay within 80 or 90 percent of your child's best, asthma is in good control. But if there are frequent dips below 80 percent, you need to see the doctor. Either your child's asthma isn't well controlled or he or she isn't giving a consistent effort.

The change in peak flow after quick-relief medication is important to know. Check peak flows before and after giving quick-relief medicine.

If the peak flow starts low then improves dramatically, it means that the muscle around the breathing tube was squeezing tightly (probably stimulated by some inflammation). On the other hand, if your child's peak flow remains low after using the quick-relief medication, then there may be much more of a problem. The most likely reason for the flow remaining low is that inflammation has caused the breathing tubes to swell. Other possibilities include poor technique in use of the inhaler or peak flow meter, or difficulty breathing due to an illness other than asthma.

CHEATING ON A PEAK FLOW METER

It's easy to cheat on the peak flow meter. I didn't learn about cheating from a book or from my professors. I learned about it from my patients. It is not that the child is trying to be bad or to get away with something. Children want to get their best numbers. And they can figure out ways to get the meter reading higher that have nothing to do with their lung function.

Most kids will figure out how to cheat on the meter fairly quickly. Most parents take a little longer to catch up. The "instructions" on cheating below are given to help parents keep one step ahead of their kids.

It is important to recognize cheating, because if your child cheats, the number she gets for her peak flow has nothing to do with lung function and tells you nothing about her asthma.

Cheating to Get a "Too High" Peak Flow
There are several ways to get a "too high" peak flow. One is to cough into the meter. Another is to build pressure in the mouth, then suddenly release it—what I call the "chipmunk maneuver." For the Assess peak flow meter, putting a finger over the hole in the back will also send the indicator way too high.

Cheating to Get a "Too Low" Peak Flow
This is even easier. If your child doesn't breathe in all the way and doesn't put maximum effort into it, the peak flow number will make you think things are worse than they really are. Sometimes a parent needs to be a bit of a cheerleader or coach to get the best effort out of a child.

If your child starts blowing before he puts the meter into the mouth, the resulting number will also underestimate true lung function.

I think it's best to check peak flows once or twice a day. That way it becomes part of a daily routine. But some families don't like the imposition of checking peak flow rates every day. I advise them to check peak flow rates at least once a week or so. Increase it to two to three times a day if the child has a runny nose, scratchy throat, cough, wheeze, chest tightness, or other cause for concern.

The peak flow meter is a great tool for sorting out breathing symptoms. Is the cough from a cold, from allergies, or from asthma? Are the breathing tubes open or are they starting to close down? How much have they closed down? Check the peak flow! A head cold won't cause a low peak flow, because it affects the nasal passages, not the breathing tubes.

Incidentally, the peak flow meter has saved parents a lot of arguing with their kids over asthma. For example, children who want to go out and play with friends will say they feel fine. Maybe they do, maybe they're in denial, or maybe they just want to go out and play. The peak flow meter is a great way to see if they're right.

Keeping an Asthma Diary

Rather than trying to keep track of daily peak flows in your head, keep a diary. There are so many important things in life to pay attention to that we really can't remember what our peak flows have been. Do you remember what you had for dinner fourteen nights ago?

A diary lets you see trends. Write down in addition what medicine your child takes and when it is taken. Write down any new activities or changes that might affect asthma—for example, sleepovers.

You may even be able to identify some of your child's asthma triggers. If one morning she visits her friend with the cat, and that evening her peak flows are down, you have identified a likely asthma trigger.

A diary is a big help for the doctor, too. Now instead of just the brief time available for the office visit, the doctor has several weeks (or months) of data, and can use it to make a much better assessment of what you need to do to control your child's asthma.

There are many excellent ways to keep an asthma diary. Some people like using a calendar, others a sheet of graph paper. The computer-savvy among us may use a spreadsheet or database program (such as Microsoft Excel or Access). The minimum information that an asthma diary should have is the date, time, and peak flow reading. Ideally, it should also include medications taken, and space to write in exposure to potential asthma triggers or changes in daily routine. It is often helpful if there is a way to tell if the peak flow is in the green, yellow, or red zone. I have provided a sample diary form in appendix A.

Alternatives to the Peak Flow Meter

Peak flow monitoring isn't for everyone. Most children under five years of age cannot perform peak flows reliably. Some older kids have trouble putting in a consistent effort. Some families find it too much of an inconvenience.

For these families, we work to help the children and their parents identify and sort out early symptoms. That approach isn't as reliable as peak flow monitoring, but it's a whole lot better than waiting for a crisis.

We look at four types of symptoms:

1. Symptoms that are *directly* related to tightness of the breathing tube. These include:
   - Tickle in the throat
   - Dry cough
   - Chest tightness and/or chest pain

- Wheezing (a high-pitched musical sound, almost like a whistle in the chest)
- Fast breathing

2. Symptoms that are related to *conditions* that can lead to a flare-up, such as allergies or a cold. Some of the most common include:
   - Allergies: itchy, red eyes, runny nose
   - Colds: runny nose and fever
   - Ear infections: ear pain, nausea, vomiting, fever
   - Sinus infections: greenish-yellow discharge from the nose that does not go away after a week or more (a few days of greenish-yellow nasal discharge is normal after a cold)

3. Symptoms that signal moderate to severe difficulty breathing. *If these symptoms are present, your child needs emergency medical attention.* If your doctor or urgent care clinic is nearby, is equipped to handle emergencies, and can see you right away, that may be an appropriate source of care. Otherwise, go to the nearest emergency room. These symptoms include:
   - Difficulty sleeping due to difficulty breathing (the body values breathing over sleeping)
   - In infants, difficulty feeding due to difficulty breathing (again, breathing takes priority)
   - Sucking in of the chest and/or belly with each breath (doctors call this "retractions")
   - Nostrils widening with each breath
   - Fast breathing at rest

4. Symptoms that signal severe difficulty breathing. *If you see these signs, call 911 immediately. There is a high risk of death if immediate action is not taken.* Severe symptoms include:
   - Breathing so hard that it is difficult to walk or talk
   - A hunched-over posture, trying to use every muscle in the body to breathe
   - Lips and/or fingers turning blue
   - A look of severe anxiety and/or agitation because it has become extremely difficult to get air in or out

Reading the Signs

Usually the first sign to show up in a flare-up is an occasional cough, a slight tickle in the throat, maybe a slight wheeze. As the flare-up gets established, sleeping becomes difficult. Breathing becomes more rapid. Your child may feel chest pain or chest tightness. You may notice your child starting to slow down. Coughing or wheezing progress from occasional to persistent. Quick-relief medicine doesn't seem to last as long or work as well.

When I'm admitting a child to the hospital for asthma in the wee hours, I will often ask the parents how the child felt the day before. I often hear that the child didn't sleep well, and needed his quick-relief inhaler or breathing treatments several times through the night. Or they will tell me that she spent much of the day coughing. These signs would get my attention as a parent.

The symptoms tend to happen on a sliding scale—subtle at first, then growing more noticeable as the flare-up worsens. But sometimes the symptoms can fool you.

For example, some people think that wheezing always accompanies an asthma flare-up. I had one doctor call me from the emergency room about a patient who had trouble breathing but wasn't wheezing. The doctor knew something was wrong, but she was convinced it wasn't asthma.

Yet when we started aggressive asthma treatment, the patient began to feel a bit better, her breathing tubes started to open up—and she started wheezing! The breathing tubes had finally opened up enough so that air could move through them and generate a wheeze.

Many parents develop a sort of radar that can pick up on signs early. Sometimes there is just a gut feeling that something's wrong. In my experience, if parents sense a problem, they're often right.

Breathing Rates

In an asthma flare-up, breathing gets faster as the lungs work to shuttle air through ever-narrower passages. Of course, activity or excitement will cause breathing to speed up, too. So it's best to measure the breathing rate when your child is at rest.

The breathing rate is simply the number of breaths taken in one minute. Count the number of breaths your child takes in a full 60 seconds. (Resist the urge to count for 15 seconds and multiply by four, your result may be inaccurate. Breathing patterns, especially in young children, tend to be a bit irregular.)

When a child is breathing hard with asthma, it's a little tricky to tell what counts as a full breath. Here are three good methods:

1. Watch the chest move up and down with each breath.
2. Listen to the chest to hear the air move in and out with each breath.
3. Place a moistened finger under your child's nose to feel the air movement as he or she exhales.

Normal breathing rates are as follows:

- For an infant: 20 to 40 breaths per minute
- For a toddler: 18 to 30 breaths per minute
- For a school-age child: 16 to 25 breaths per minute

Managing Asthma Flare-Ups

In the next chapter, we'll show you in detail how you and your doctor can use these measurements to create a tailored plan for managing flare-ups. But the essential principle is to *use quick-relief medications to open up the airways quickly,* and to *take steps to get the inflammation under control.*

Sometimes, if asthma symptoms are mild and occasional, a puff or two of a quick-relief medication is enough to make your child feel better. You may need to increase the doses of inhaled corticosteroids for a week or two to control the low-grade inflammation.

If the flare-up is more severe, you need to take more aggressive steps—for example, using higher doses of quick-relief medicine plus a few days of an oral corticosteroid to control the advanced inflammation.

Both are critical. The quick-relief medications provide only a few hours of symptom relief. They don't get to the underlying problem—the inflammation. But you need them to buy time until the oral corticosteroids (like prednisone) start working. This one-two punch may be enough to keep a moderate flare-up from becoming a severe one.[2]

Let's go on to take a closer look at the medications that we use.

Quick-Relief Medications

Quick-relief medicines relax the muscle layer that surrounds the breathing tubes. When inhaled, their action kicks in within minutes; however, their effect lasts only for a few hours.

Quick-relief medicines do nothing for the swelling and inflammation that drive the asthma flare-up. They only treat symptoms. Using quick-relief medicine *alone* for treatment of a moderate to severe asthma flare-up is like painting over rust—it just hides the underlying problem.

Different doctors have different preferences, but I will give you my own views on the pros and cons of each. Of course, decisions about medicines should always be discussed with your doctor.

Albuterol (Ventolin, Ventolin Rotocaps, Proventil, Proventil HFA)

What this drug is: Perhaps the most popular quick-relief asthma medicine is albuterol. It comes as a metered-dose inhaler, dry powder inhaler, solution for nebulizer, oral syrup, tablets, and extended-release tablets.

When inhaled, albuterol quickly relieves asthma symptoms. It acts by relaxing the muscle surrounding the breathing tubes (hence the other term for this class of medicine, bronchodilator). It starts acting within minutes; however, the effects wear off after about four hours.

Albuterol can also be taken by mouth. Though this route may be more convenient, a couple of hours may pass before the effects peak. It has to get from the stomach to the bloodstream then on to the lungs. As only a small part of the medicine gets to the lungs, the benefit of oral albuterol is often less than that of inhaled albuterol. Albuterol taken by mouth can work for mild asthma symptoms. It does not get enough medicine to the lungs for relief of moderate to severe asthma symptoms.

Side effects of albuterol are generally minimal, but can include stimulation (nervousness), rapid heart rate, and headaches.

What I like about it: My preferred quick-relief medication is the albuterol metered-dose inhaler. It is effective, inexpensive, easy to use, and fast acting. The benefit is improved and side effects reduced when it is used with a spacer device.

Medication from a metered-dose inhaler can be easily and quickly given to an infant or young child using a spacer with mask, such as the AeroChamber with Mask.

Using multiple puffs of albuterol from a metered-dose inhaler is an effective, inexpensive, and convenient alternative to using a nebulizer machine when higher doses of albuterol are needed.

The Proventil HFA preparation is more expensive than other albuterol inhalers. What you pay for is the absence of chlorofluorocarbon (CFC) propellant.

Albuterol dry powder inhalers are small and convenient to use. Inhalation is totally powered by the breath, so chlorofluorocarbon (CFC) propellants are not needed.

A nebulizer (see chapter 5) is a machine that aerosolizes liquid medicine into a mist that is inhaled over about 15 minutes. It doesn't require coordination between puffing and breathing. Very high doses of albuterol may be easier to administer via nebulizer.

Albuterol syrup is easy to administer to an infant who is having only mild asthma symptoms.

What I don't like about it: In albuterol metered-dose inhalers chlorofluorocarbons (CFCs) are used as the propellant (except in the Proventil HFA preparation).

Albuterol dry powder inhalers cannot be used by young children because you need to be able to take a rapid, deep breath and hold it. Some people may be unable to use the dry powder inhaler during a moderate to severe asthma flare-up, when getting air in is difficult.

Albuterol via nebulizer machine requires an expensive, bulky machine to administer. It takes about 15 minutes or so to give a breathing treatment.

Albuterol syrup or pills are less effective and have more side effects than inhaled albuterol. They also take longer to work than inhaled albuterol.

Levalbulterol (Xenopex)

Xenopex is a preparation of albuterol for the nebulizer. The manufacturer claims that because it has only the active part of albuterol, it causes slightly fewer side effects. Regular albuterol generally is well tolerated, and I'm not sure that the increased cost is worth the small bene-fit. Furthermore, it only comes in a formulation for the nebulizer.

Terbutaline (Brethaire)

Terbutaline is similar to albuterol; however, it is much more expensive. For this reason, it is not commonly used outside of the hospital.[3] As an inhaler, it has no advantages over albuterol.

Pirbuterol (Maxair, Maxair Autohaler)

What this drug is: Pirbuterol is a lot like albuterol in its properties and actions as a quick reliever. The niche that this medication has is the "autohaler" technology. The autohaler automatically releases a dose of medicine as you start to inhale. This feature makes it easier to coordinate release of the medicine with breathing in.

What I like about it: The autohaler technology makes coordination of the breath with the puff from the inhaler a whole lot easier.

What I don't like about it: It's expensive. It can't be used with a spacer device. Some people (myself included) have a tendency to stop breathing in once the burst of medicine hits the back of the throat.

In a severe asthma attack, it may be difficult to inhale with sufficient force to trigger the inhaler to release medicine.

Maxair Autohaler cannot be used by young children.

Metaproterenol (Alupent, Metaprel)

Metaproterenol is a quick reliever that was frequently used before albuterol came on the market. It has more side effects than albuterol, so it no longer widely used. *I would avoid metaproterenol, as much better alternatives are available.*

Isoproterenol (Isuprel, Medihaler-Iso)

Isoproterenol acts quickly, but the effects don't last long. Because of its potential for cardiac toxicity (heart injury), it is rarely used now. Deaths have been caused from excessive use of this medication. *I do not recommend its use.*

Epinephrine (Primatene Mist)

Though Primatene Mist is quick acting and available over the counter, what the advertisements don't tell you is that it has a very short duration of action. Side effects are much greater than with the prescription asthma inhalers. Though I could see using this medicine fifty years ago when there wasn't anything better available, *there is no good reason to use it currently.*

NO SYMPTOMS, NO PROBLEM? NO WAY!

Quick-relief medications are sometimes *too* effective. One of the most common reasons that kids end up in emergency rooms is that parents thought the crisis had passed when it hadn't. The bronchodilators are to blame.

Here's the problem: Bronchodilators like albuterol do such a great job of relieving symptoms that your child looks and feels great. But these drugs have no effect on the underlying problem.

Flare-ups are fundamentally driven by inflammation of the breathing tubes. Bronchodilators work by relaxing the muscle. And when they wear off—as they inevitably do within a few hours—you're right back where you started.

Or, to be more accurate, you may be *worse* off than when you started, because the inflammation has been smoldering for another four to six hours.

Don't let these drugs lull you into a false sense of security. If your child is experiencing a moderate or severe flare-up, he or she needs to be treated with oral corticosteroids—the sooner the better.

I don't want to suggest that bronchodilators are somehow bad or shouldn't be used. They're superb at what they do, which is quickly getting the breathing tubes open. The problem is that they only do half the job, and only temporarily.

In a moderate to severe asthma flare-up, you need to treat *both* the inflammation (causing swelling of the breathing tube) and the bronchospasm (the tightening of the muscle around the breathing tubes).

Reversing Swelling and Inflammation:
Oral Corticosteroids

Oral corticosteroids are powerful medicines used to shrink the swelling and inflammation that drive the asthma flare-up. They take about six to eight hours to start working, so the sooner they're started, the easier the flare-up will be to reverse.

Nighttime tends to be the worst time for people with asthma. Lung function is normally at its lowest in the middle of the night. Studies have shown that an oral corticosteroid dose given in the midafternoon will help a child with an asthma flare-up get through the night better. If you give the dose at 3 P.M., it will be kicking in solidly by the time your child is asleep at night.[4]

Side effects from oral corticosteroids are common. The most common are mood changes, increased appetite, weight gain, and suppression of fever. Children who are exposed to or develop chicken pox while on oral corticosteroids can develop a severe case (a good reason to get your child vaccinated now if you haven't already).

Generally the most severe corticosteroid side effects aren't seen with the short, occasional bursts that we use to control flare-ups. The big problems with side effects occur when you use these drugs daily for months or years. Then it can weaken bones, thin the skin, increase susceptibility to infection, cause cataracts, make you more susceptible to bruising, suppress growth, and increase the risk for stomach ulcers.

As a rough guide, I consider a "short burst" to be five days or less, and "occasional" as less than four times per year. If your child needs oral corticosteroids more often then this, talk with your doctor, as your asthma management plan may need to be changed.

Following are some of the pros and cons of the different oral corticosteroid medicines on the market in the United States.

Prednisone

Prednisone is one of the most commonly used corticosteroid preparations on the market. Because it's an older medication, inexpensive generic preparations are available.

What I like about it: It's effective, widely used, and inexpensive.

What I don't like about it: Its bad taste; prednisone syrup is extremely bitter and unpalatable. I have a hard time getting kids to take it. The pills are fine—if swallowed quickly and not crushed or chewed.

Prednisolone (Prelone, Pediapred)

Prednisolone is an oral corticosteroid that is very similar to prednisone. The advantage of prednisolone is that it does not taste quite as bad as prednisone, so I use it for children who need a liquid (syrup) preparation.

Prelone liquid (15 mg per 5 ml) is more concentrated than Pediapred (5 mg per 5 ml). On the plus side, it means less for your child to swallow. On the downside, the taste is worse.

Pediapred liquid is only one-third as concentrated as Prelone. At about the same price per volume, this comes out to three times the cost for amount of drug delivered. The benefit of Pediapred, however, is that the taste is not offensive. I have seen some children who adamantly refuse Prelone willingly take Pediapred.

What I like about it: Compared to Pediapred, Prelone is less expensive and a smaller volume of medicine needs to be given.

The taste of Pediapred is not offensive. This makes it easier to give to some children.

What I don't like about it: Prelone has a bitter taste and Pediapred is expensive.

Methylprednisolone (Medrol, Solumedrol)

Methylprednisolone is very similar to prednisone, but more expensive. There is no advantage or disadvantage to using this medication compared to prednisone or prednisolone. Methylprednisolone is commonly used in the hospital when an intravenous corticosteroid is needed.

Dexamethasone (Decadron)

A single dose of dexamethasone will last about two to three times longer than the other corticosteroid preparations. If your child has a hard time taking medicines, this may be an advantage. Because of the increased risk for side effects that comes with the increased duration of action, this medicine is generally not my first choice.

What I like about it: It has a longer duration of action than prednisone or methylprednisolone, and it can be given as an injection if the child is vomiting and unable to take medicine by mouth.

What I don't like about it: The longer duration of action increases the risk of side effects.

Following Up

The last—and often overlooked—step in managing a flare-up is the follow-up. Did the flare-up get resolved completely? Do we know why it happened and how it might be prevented in the future? Are there triggers that can be controlled? Early signs that were missed? Is your child taking the preventive medication? Using the inhaler correctly? Is the dose too low? Too high? Can it be stepped down—that is, reduced gradually?

When I was studying lung disease in New Orleans, part of my research involved investigating why children with asthma came into the Charity Hospital Emergency Room. Surprisingly, I found that most patients loved the emergency room! When they had an asthma attack they could come in and get taken care of right away. They got excellent treatment—but it was for the attack. What they didn't get, by and large, was follow-up and a plan for preventive care. That meant they lived from crisis to crisis—and were probably going to be seen again, and soon, in the emergency room.[5] One of the most important parts of managing flare-ups is to *prevent the next one from happening*!

Managing Flare-Ups: Common Problems and Solutions

Here are some of the problems and concerns that we see in our practice, along with some ideas on how to address them:

By the time I get to the doctor the flare-up is already out of control.

- Discuss with your doctor having an emergency supply of prednisone (or prednisolone) on hand at home. The earlier you start working on the inflammation, the easier it will be to conquer.

- Maybe your "red zone" threshold—the peak flow rate your doctor has set as the signal that a flare-up is starting—is set too low for your child (see next chapter). Discuss with your doctor having a higher red zone. I usually use 50 to 60 percent of personal best peak flow as the threshold, but I had one patient whose flare-ups progressed very rapidly. We decided to start prednisone when her peak flow hit 70 percent of her personal best—and she's done much better since.
- Know what's likely to trigger a flare-up. Some kids always get severe asthma flare-ups when they get a cold. For these patients, starting prednisone at the first sign of the cold will help.[6] I don't recommend this step for most patients, as it may lead to taking a lot of prednisone. But if the asthma is so bad that the alternative is ending up in the ER or hospital on lots of corticosteroids anyway, this may be the better choice.

My child's asthma flare-up is still not well controlled, even after several days on prednisone.

- Think about what else could be keeping the flare-up going. Sinus infections are a common culprit when an asthma flare-up doesn't get better.
- Consider whether a new asthma trigger has been brought into the home—for example, a visiting relative who smokes, a fireplace you have just started to use, a Christmas tree, a new pet, etc.
- See your doctor. It is important to figure out what is going on and to treat it if possible.

My child is having lots of asthma flare-ups, so she needs lots of prednisone. I'm worried about side effects.

- If your child is having lots of asthma flare-ups, take a harder look at the first two lines of defense—managing the environment and managing the breathing tubes. Be more aggressive about controlling your child's environment. For example, find out whether he or she is being exposed to smoke outside your home—say, at a friend's house or in a carpool. You may have to insist that the kids play at your house or pull out of the carpool if other drivers insist on smoking. But it's your child's health at stake.

- If you've already taken care of the basics, such as using a daily preventive medication and controlling asthma triggers in the home, it may be time to see an asthma specialist (pediatric pulmonologist or allergist) to help you figure out what's going on.

9

Putting It All Together:
How to Create an Asthma
Self-Management Plan

Twenty years ago, doctors like Guillermo Mendoza saw a problem.

Doctors were just learning about all of the things we've been talking about—the importance of using long-acting inhaled anti-inflammatory medicine (such as the inhaled corticosteroids) to prevent asthma, the need to monitor flare-ups and act on them early, the delicate balance between short-acting bronchodilators and oral corticosteroids.

That was a lot to keep track of, even for doctors. So how on earth could patients—especially children—keep it all straight?

The particular problem that Dr. Mendoza was grappling with was helping kids know which medications to take and when. He and others started experimenting with color-coding the medications—for example, green medications for preventive medications; yellow medications to use when a flare-up was starting; and red medications to bring a crisis under control.

For a variety of reasons, that scheme didn't work out. But the idea of a green, yellow, and red zone system for managing asthma stuck. Even kids who are too young to read get the idea that green means safe, yellow means caution, and red means danger.

Eventually, these and similar efforts evolved into an intuitive way to teach kids about their asthma and help them sort out all of this complex information.

Now the green-yellow-red system for managing asthma is officially endorsed by the National Asthma Education and Prevention Program (NAEPP) and is used all over the world. It's a cornerstone of our program at Kaiser Permanente as well.

There are a lot of variations on the basic idea. I'll tell you in this chapter how we use it to help families put all this complex information into a self-management plan they can use every day.

Here's the idea in a nutshell:

1. We use the peak flow meter as our basic measuring tool (see chapter 8 for more information on peak flow monitoring).

2. Using findings from the child's history and physical examination, we establish three zones of peak flow measurements.

3. The *green zone* means "safe." As long as the child's peak flow readings are within this zone, we know that the asthma is well controlled. We maintain the preventive medications (inhaled corticosteroids). We expect that the child will need bronchodilators (quick relievers) only occasionally—for example, before exercise, or when he is exposed to an unusually high level of pollen in the air.

4. The *yellow zone* means "caution." The yellow zone consists of peak flow readings that are somewhat lower than the best effort, but not dramatically so. For example, if a child's best peak flow reading is 300, the yellow zone might range from 150 to 250. Those figures aren't carved in stone; we try to tailor the zone based on what we know about the child's history and how consistent their peak flows are when they are well, and we may adjust it as we see what happens going forward.

When a child's peak flow reading is in the yellow zone, the breathing tubes have started to narrow. The child and parent know to adjust their medications to bring their asthma back in control.

5. The *red zone* means "danger." When peak flow readings fall into this zone, an asthma flare-up has taken hold. This is a warning signal. Prompt aggressive action needs to be taken.

The power of this system is its simplicity. It relies on one measurement: the peak flow reading. Parents and kids have to keep track of only two numbers: the thresholds for the yellow and red zones. As long as they stay in green, the rules are simple: keep taking the medications as prescribed. If they move into the other zones, they have a simple written form (suitable for framing on the refrigerator) that reminds them what to do.

One such form is illustrated on page 120.[1] Other forms can be found as part of the National Asthma Education and Prevention Program (NAEPP) asthma care guideline.[2]

Alternatives to Daily Peak Flow Monitoring

In my practice I have found that not everyone is able—or willing—to do daily peak flow monitoring. Children younger than five or six years generally are not able to do accurate or reproducible peak flows. Asthma symptoms can be used as a guide to determine green, yellow, and red zones. However, just like using a thermometer to determine the fever when a child feels warm, the peak flow is the best home measure of breathing tube tightness.

Another acceptable approach is to check the peak flow every one to two weeks. This keeps up your child's skills using the peak flow meter and keeps you on top of what his or her best peak flow rate is. In this way, growth doesn't catch you by surprise.

If you use this approach, you need to go back to checking peak flows twice a day when there are signs of potential problems, such as wheezing, chest tightness, runny nose, or so on.

Checking and recording peak flows for a couple of weeks before a doctor's visit helps your doctor to see how well (or poorly) controlled your child's asthma has been over time. This lets your doctor know if a more aggressive approach to asthma control is needed or if dosages can be cut back.

Creating an Individualized Plan

The specifics of this approach must be tailored to each individual. For example, the peak flow values that we use to set the green, yellow, and red zones will vary from child to child. We start with some general ballpark figures, but we tailor them based on experience. For example, if flare-ups tend to progress quickly, we'd likely set the red zone higher so we have more time to take action.

The same goes for the medications. Depending on a variety of factors—the severity of the asthma, the child's response to different medications, and so on—we come up with a tailored response for each zone.

Keep in mind that controlling asthma triggers in the environment should be the first part of any plan. The fewer triggers, the less medication your child will need.

Of course, your written green/yellow/red zone plan should be designed in partnership with your doctor. But if you know how to construct an asthma management plan, you can be a more effective partner. Following are some guidelines and examples of actual plans we've developed to give you an idea of the issues to consider.

Guidelines for the Green Zone

Finding Your Child's Green Zone

By peak flows: In the green zone, asthma is well controlled. That means that the lung function is normal. Peak flows are at least 80 to 90 percent of your child's personal best.

When is it appropriate to use 90 percent, and when should we use the more liberal 80 percent cutoff for the green zone? Monitor and chart your child's peak flow every day when asthma is in good control. If peak flow is usually within 90 percent of personal best—that is, less than 10 percent variability—when he's doing well, use that figure as the cutoff. Anything less suggests that the asthma is starting to flare up.

Some children's peak flows bounce around a little more even when they're healthy. So if your child's peak flow ranges between 80 and 100 percent of personal best (20 percent variability) when her asthma is in control, use the 80 percent cutoff. The principle is simple: Know what's normal for your child. Dips below that level are signs of trouble.

Now, regardless of variability, 80 percent is about the lowest you should go for the green zone threshold. Ten to 20 percent variability in peak flow can be normal. If peak flows fluctuate more than that, there could be a problem. Either your child's asthma is not well controlled, or there's a problem with the peak flow technique. If peak flow rate regularly goes below 80 percent of your child's personal best, bring this to the attention of your doctor.

Where should your child's personal best peak flow be? Peak flow rates, like lung size, vary by how tall the child is. If you know your child's height, you can look up a predicted peak flow (see the table of average peak flow rates in appendix B). Keep in mind that the "normal" peak flow only represents an average value for children of that height. Your child may have a personal best peak flow that is either above or below predicted. However, when the personal best peak flow rate is not known, the predicted peak flow gives us a good place to start.

By symptoms: In the green zone, there should be no asthma symptoms—no cough, no wheeze, no chest tightness. The breathing rate is normal. Normal breathing rates for children at rest are as follows:

> 20–40 breaths per minute for an infant
> 18–30 breaths per minute for a toddler
> 16–25 breaths per minute for a school-age child

Green Zone Tips

The goal is to stay in the green zone every day, and to get back there quickly if there is a lapse into the yellow or red zones.

If you find your child frequently bouncing in and out of the yellow (or red) zone, you need to see your health care provider to reevaluate the green zone plan.

Conversely, if a high dose of medication has kept your child rock solid stable at the top of his or her green zone, maybe it's time to talk to your doctor about slowly stepping down the dose of preventive medicine.

See the section "Staying in the Green Zone," on page 108, for a green zone medication plan.

Guidelines for the Yellow Zone

Finding Your Child's Yellow Zone

By peak flows: The yellow zone consists of peak flow readings that are somewhat lower than best effort, but not dramatically so.

We usually set the upper cutoff of the yellow zone at 80 to 90 percent of personal best peak flow, the lower end at 50 to 60 percent. For example, if the personal best peak flow reading is 300, the yellow zone might range from 150 to 240. Those figures aren't carved in stone; we try to tailor the zone based on what we know about the patient's past history and may adjust it as we see what happens going forward.

By symptoms: In the yellow zone, there may be very mild asthma symptoms, such as a slight cough, mild wheeze, or slight chest tightness. The breathing rate at rest may be near the upper limits of normal (see normal breathing rates above). However, sometimes in the yellow zone there may be no symptoms at all, only a decreased peak flow rate.

Yellow Zone Tips

The yellow zone means caution. A flare-up is in its earliest stages. Asthma flare-ups are like weeds—the sooner you root them out, the better. So take action upon entering the yellow zone, and monitor closely to see the response. Is your child heading back to the green zone? Or are things diving toward the red zone?

The yellow zone requires caution. Just like a yellow traffic light, it tells you this is a place you should only be in briefly. If your child is stuck in the yellow zone, or bouncing in and out of it frequently, it's time to see your health care provider. The asthma is not in good control.

Yellow Zone Medication Plans

- *Add a quick-relief medicine (such as albuterol).* The exact medicine choice and dose should be discussed with you child's doctor and individualized to your child's needs. My usual practice for most patients is to start the albuterol metered-dose inhaler (given via spacer device) at 2 puffs every 4 to 6 hours.

- *Increase preventive (inhaled corticosteroid) medicine.* I will usually increase the dose of an inhaled corticosteroid by 25 to 50 percent. I will continue this higher dose for not more than one to two weeks. If a child is stuck in the yellow zone for that long, there is a problem that needs to be looked into by a doctor. Of course, medication plans should *always* be discussed with your child's doctor.

   Certain medications should NOT have their dose increased for yellow or red zones. *Do NOT increase the dose of theophylline (SloBid, TheoDur, Uniphyl), salmeterol (Serevent), or leukotriene modifiers (Accolate, Singulair).*

- If your child doesn't get better soon (two to three days), see a doctor to find out what is going on.

Guidelines for the Red Zone

Finding Your Child's Red Zone

By peak flows: Your child is in the red zone if peak flow drops below 50 or 60 percent of personal best (even if it improves after taking quick-relief medication).

How do we decide whether to use 50 or 60 percent as the red zone cutoff? It depends on the previous history of asthma severity. If there's a history of severe flare-ups needing hospitalization or emergency room visits, it's best to take aggressive action earlier, so I use 60 percent of personal best (that is, a 40 percent drop) as the red zone cutoff. If asthma has been mild and rock solid stable, I'm more comfortable waiting until the peak flow has dropped to 50 percent of personal best before taking aggressive action.

By symptoms: You may see persistent or frequent coughing, wheezing, rapid breathing, or chest tightness. There may be sucking in of the skin between the ribs or below the chest. There may be difficulty sleeping because of the trouble breathing.

In the red zone, the breathing rate at rest is rapid:

- More than 50 breaths per minute for an infant
- More than 40 breaths per minute for a toddler
- More than 30 breaths per minute for a school-age child

Keep in mind that every child is unique. Few will show every one of these symptoms when they are in their red zone. In fact, most children will show only one or two of these signs when they first enter the red zone, with more being present the deeper they get. Be alert, and get to know your child's first signs of moderate to severe asthma.

Red Zone Tips

The red zone means danger. When peak flow readings fall into this zone, a flare-up has taken root. About half of your child's lung function has been lost. Entering the red zone means that your child is not far away from big trouble. You need to take immediate action and see the doctor.

Red Zone Medication Plans

To reverse the inflammation, we use a powerful oral corticosteroid medication, such as prednisone or prednisolone. The earlier you start, the easier it will be to reverse the flare-up and the less medicine your child will end up needing. These medicines usually take about six to eight hours for their effects to kick in.

To relax the grip of the squeezing muscle, your child will also need to use a quick-relief inhaler like albuterol. Often a higher dose than usual is needed.

To prevent relapse back into the red zone, the dose of preventive medication may need to be increased.

If your child is in the red zone, *see your doctor* to find out what the trigger is and if additional medication is needed.

See chapter 8, "Managing Flare-Ups," for more information on what to do in the red zone.

A WORD ABOUT ORAL CORTICOSTEROID BURSTS

Oral corticosteroids like prednisone are powerful medications. They can have significant side effects, but there's nothing like them to reverse the swelling and inflammation that drives a moderate to severe asthma flare-up.

Out of concern for side effects, many people try to wait as long as possible into a flare-up to start prednisone. That is often a recipe for using more—not less. The more advanced the inflammation is, the more difficult it is to reverse. If you start early, one to two days of therapy may have your child back in the green zone. Wait, and you may face a 2 A.M. emergency room visit, hospitalization, and a week of prednisone to fix the damage.

If your child needs prednisone, let your doctor know sooner rather than later. But if you know it's needed, don't hesitate to start it at home. It gives you that much more of a jump on getting the asthma under control.

Staying in the Green Zone

The ultimate goal of asthma self-management is to stay in the green zone.

Probably one of the most challenging parts of asthma management is finding a green zone plan that works well—using neither too little nor too much medicine. The green zone plan usually reflects the severity of the underlying asthma.

If there's only a little bit of inflammation and it happens only occasionally, you don't need to do too much to control the asthma. But if there is lots of inflammation in the breathing tubes nearly all the time, then control is more difficult.

To create a tailored green zone plan, first decide, from the descriptions that follow, which category of severity your child's asthma falls into:

- Mild intermittent
- Mild persistent
- Moderate persistent
- Severe persistent

Some people fall outside of these classifications altogether. We'll show you what to do in those cases as well.

Mild Intermittent Asthma

In this category, asthma symptoms are occasional, mild, and don't last for long. You shouldn't see asthma symptoms (cough, wheeze, or chest tightness) more than twice a week, nor should your child need quick-relief medications any more often than that. Most of the time your child should feel completely well. A quick-relief inhaler should last four to six months or more before running out.

Generally, children with mild intermittent asthma don't need hospitalizations or emergency room visits.

The peak flow rate can help you determine if asthma is intermittent or persistent. Check your child's peak flow two to three times a day for several weeks. If the peak flow stays within 10 to 20 percent of personal best (without medication), asthma is intermittent. If the peak flow fluctuates more than 20 percent over that period, asthma may be persistent; fluctuating peak flows mean that the breathing tubes are tightening and opening. This pattern suggests that the asthma never quite fully goes away, even if symptoms disappear.

Medication guidelines: If asthma is truly intermittent, most of the time your child will be staying in the green zone without any medicine. Those brief occasions when there is a dip to the yellow zone should resolve with just a little bit of quick-relief medication. If your child's asthma is truly mild and intermittent, the inflammation of the breathing tubes will go away on its own after a day or two.

A person with intermittent asthma can have a severe flare-up to red zone—or worse, needing more aggressive treatment, including oral corticosteroids. Be attentive to what is happening in your child's body.

Mild Persistent Asthma

Here asthma episodes are brief but frequent. They're easily relieved by use of quick-relief medicines. There may be coughing or wheezing twice a week or more, but not every day. Sleep may be interrupted twice a month or more, but not every week. Peak flow rates may frequently dip to 70 to 80 percent of best, but they don't go below 70 percent. Lung function measured in a doctor's office, however, may be completely normal.

Though the consequences of mild persistent asthma may be easily controlled with quick-relief medicine, there is likely ongoing, persistent inflammation of the breathing tubes—which, as we've seen, can cause permanent damage. In addition, the ongoing daily smolder of inflammation creates a higher risk of flare-up.

Medication guidelines: If asthma symptoms are mild but frequent, it's usually best to use medicine every day.

A low dose of an inhaled corticosteroid medication is often most effective, easiest to use, and least expensive. Depending on which inhaled steroid preparation you choose, generally a dose of one to two puffs, once or twice a day, should be sufficient.

Chromone (cromolyn = Intal, nedocromil = Tilade) medication is another option. Your child will need to use it more often. These medicines are most effective when used three to four times a day, every day.

Some people with mild persistent asthma will do well on a leukotriene modifier medication (montelukast = Singulair or zafirlukast = Accolate).

Which medicine is right for your child? Cromolyn and nedocromil have an excellent record of safety but are inconvenient and expensive. Low-dose inhaled corticosteroids have minimal side effects and are cheaper and more convenient.

Moderate Persistent Asthma

With moderate persistent asthma, you'll notice daily asthma symptoms. Quick-relief medicine is needed just about every day. Sleep may be interrupted once a week or more. Exercise may be difficult. Lung function measured in a doctor's office is mildly abnormal. Peak flow rates may often drop as low as 60 percent of personal best. Your child probably misses many school days because of asthma.

With moderate persistent asthma, there is significant ongoing inflammation of the breathing tubes. There's a high risk for asthma attacks— severe enough to require emergency room treatment or hospitalization.

Medication options. For moderate asthma, weak anti-inflammatory medicines like cromolyn and nedocromil probably aren't going to be strong enough to do the job. Your child will probably need a moderate dose of an inhaled corticosteroid medication. Start with enough to get the asthma in control; then, every month or so, in teamwork with your doctor, work to find the lowest dose that will keep it there. A typical starting dose for a child is 200 to 400 micrograms per day. Don't make changes more often than once a month, because it takes that long for the drugs to work.

Sometimes a moderate dose of an inhaled corticosteroid isn't enough. In this case, your doctor may also prescribe a long-acting symptom-relieving medicine, either salmeterol (Serevent),[3] theophylline (TheoDur, SloBid, Uniphyl, others),[4] or a leukotriene modifier (Accolate, Singulair).

Severe Asthma

With severe asthma, symptoms never really go away. Coughing and shortness of breath frequently interrupt your child's sleep. He or she may go through a quick-acting symptom reliever inhaler (like albuterol) in less than a month. Peak flows are erratic. Lung function, when checked in a doctor's office, may be moderately to severely abnormal. Schoolwork probably suffers, and sports are a struggle. Your child has probably been in the hospital more than once and is on a first-name basis with emergency room staff. Your child may even have gone into an intensive care unit during a bad flare-up.

If your child has severe asthma, you have a lot to gain from getting the asthma under control. But you're going to have to put a lot of work into it. A careful search to control factors that may be triggering the asthma is important. Sometimes there are complicating medical conditions that need treatment, such as sinus infections or gastroesophageal reflux (acid reflux). Occasionally we find that the difficulty breathing is due to an illness other than asthma.[5] If your child has severe asthma, it is important to see an asthma specialist (pediatric pulmonologist or allergist).

Medication options. A moderate to high dose of an inhaled cortico-steroid is the foundation of therapy, but it's usually not enough, all by itself, to keep severe asthma well controlled. A long-acting symptom reliever (salmeterol or theophylline) is also usually needed. Sometimes a leukotriene modifier may be needed as well.

In treating severe asthma, I recommend use of a higher-potency inhaled corticosteroid such as Flovent 220 or Pulmicort. Use of these higher-potency products allows you to keep the number of puffs down to two puffs (or less) twice a day.

It is important to follow up with your child's asthma specialist. Make sure that the plan is working. Over time find the minimum medication dose needed.

Outside the Box

Sometimes asthma doesn't fit into the neat categories given above; however, we can still use the same principles of management.

A common "outside the box" category is seasonally persistent asthma (see chapter 13). If pollens are your child's major asthma trigger, his or her asthma may fit the mild intermittent category during the fall and winter but advance to moderate persistent for the spring and/or summer. The pattern may be reversed if cold viruses are your child's major asthma trigger. In these situations, you really need two green zone plans. For your child's bad season(s), use a higher dose of preventive medicine. For the good seasons, step down to a lower dose, or none at all.

Here's another outside-the-box pattern: Some people who usually do well may, once a year or so, encounter a trigger that provokes a moderate to severe flare-up. In this case, a mild intermittent asthma plan might be appropriate, but you need to be on the alert for the early signs of that asthma flare-up and use a low threshold for starting the red zone plan.

Exercise-Induced Asthma

Exercise is important for children. Have a plan for the prevention of exercise-induced asthma as part of your child's green zone plan. Usually something as simple as a puff or two of albuterol, taken just before exercise, will do the trick.

Refer to pages 51–53 for a detailed discussion of exercise-induced asthma.

What Does an Effective Asthma Plan Look Like?

Following are some examples of self-management plans that we've developed, working with kids and parents and tailoring them to the specific needs of individual patients. You can use them to get a sense of how we put the plans together and what plan might be appropriate for your child.

Let me emphasize again that the plan you and your doctor develop could look different even if your child's condition seems similar to one of these patients. The best plan will reflect not only the general principles of the zone system but your own experience.

You'll notice that one element all these plans have in common is clarity. We try to be as specific as possible about where the zones fall and what to do in each of them. That makes it easier to keep asthma under control—and it eliminates a lot of worrying and second-guessing as well.

A Plan for Mild Intermittent Asthma

Jennifer is ten years old. She has mild intermittent asthma. On most days she's fine—no coughing, no wheezing. She's a competitive runner. Vigorous exercise will cause her to cough and wheeze a little.

One of the things we note from talking to Jennifer and her parents is that she's a high achiever and very detail oriented. She follows her peak flow every day, and on most days it's within 10 percent of her personal best. Her personal best peak flow is 340 (slightly more than predicted for her age and height).

Occasionally, when she gets a cold or when the pollen count is high, she may start to cough and wheeze a little. Usually this doesn't happen more than three or four times a year.

Since we've been monitoring her asthma, she's gone into her red zone only once. Her quick-relief inhaler (albuterol) lasts for more than 6 months. Jennifer's asthma fits our definition of mild intermittent asthma.

Jennifer's Medication Plan

Personal best peak flow: 340

Green zone:
- Peak flow 300 to 340 (90 percent to 100 percent of personal best)
- No preventive medicine is needed.
- Albuterol, two puffs, is taken just before she goes out to run.

Yellow zone:
- Peak flow 170 to 300 (50 to 90 percent of best)
- Albuterol, two puffs up to four times a day, as needed

Red zone:

* Peak flow below 170 (below 50 percent of best)
* Start prednisone for a one- to five-day burst.
* Albuterol, two to six puffs every three to six hours
* See the doctor.

Jennifer is doing well with this plan. Though she has prednisone at home, she hasn't needed it. When she takes her albuterol before track meets, she does well. When she forgets it, she coughs and wheezes. Because she runs much better when she takes her medicine, her coach tries to remind her.

A Plan for Mild Persistent Asthma

Joey is eight years old. He doesn't have problems every day, but he tells me that he does have a little bit of coughing and wheezing, maybe two or three times a week. Joey's parents confirm this.

But when he catches a cold, his parents say, it's misery. He'll have a cough for a couple of weeks, sometimes longer. Exercise will also set him coughing and wheezing, especially in the winter when the air is cold and dry. When he gets like this, his quick-relief medication (albuterol) usually makes him feel better.

When I reviewed Joey's medication refills, I found that he needed to get his albuterol inhaler refilled four times in the last year.

Joey feels that his asthma isn't such a big deal, but it is "annoying," he says. It makes him feel different from other kids.

A lung function test in the office (when Joey was feeling well) was normal.

Joey's condition fits our definition of mild persistent asthma.

Joey's Medication Plan:

Personal best peak flow: 250

Green zone:

* Peak flow 200 to 250 (over 80 percent of personal best)
* Azmacort, two puffs twice daily every day

- Albuterol, two puffs before exercise (to prevent exercise induced asthma)

Joey liked the built-in spacer that comes with the Azmacort inhaler. He uses the inhaler before he goes to school and when he gets home (so he doesn't have to feel embarrassed in front of his friends and classmates).

Yellow zone:
- Peak flow 125 to 250 (50 to 80 percent of personal best)
- Albuterol, two puffs every four to six hours
- Increase Azmacort to three puffs twice a day for one to two weeks.
- If not out of yellow zone in two to three days, see a doctor.

Red zone:
- Peak flow below 125 (below 50 percent of personal best)
- Start prednisone for a one- to five-day burst.
- Albuterol, four to six puffs every three to six hours
- Azmacort, three puffs twice a day for two to three weeks
- Urgent (same day) visit with doctor

After a couple of weeks on the Azmacort Joey found that he wasn't coughing or wheezing anymore. His ability to tolerate exercise improved; now only very vigorous activity will make him cough and wheeze. By using his albuterol inhaler just before physical education, he's able to prevent even this little bit of trouble.

When he returned for follow-up after two months, we saw what a good job he had done in controlling his asthma. We were able to cut his Azmacort dose by half. He has continued to do very well on this low dose of medicine; however, if he forgets to take it for a few days, a little of that old cough and wheeze comes back.

A Plan for Moderate Asthma

Michael is twelve years old. Most days, Michael coughs and wheezes. He has trouble with physical education classes and frequently has to sit out the games. His schoolwork suffers because he is sick so often.

He goes through one albuterol inhaler a month. His mother tells me she can count on having to rush him to the emergency room at least once or twice every winter.

Michael had gotten prescriptions for corticosteroid inhalers before, but he quickly stopped using them. When I ask why, he says he forgot. Besides, the medicine tasted bad. And it didn't seem to make a difference.

Michael has moderate persistent asthma. We have had trouble getting his asthma in control because he doesn't like to use his inhaled preventive medication. Perhaps a preparation that didn't taste as bad would help. Maybe if he only had to use his medicine once a day, he would take it.

Michael's Medication Plan:

Personal best peak flow: 340

Green zone:
- Peak flow 270–340 (over 80 percent of personal best)
- Pulmicort dry powder inhaler, two puffs each morning
- Uniphyl (long-acting theophylline), one tablet each morning
- Albuterol, two puffs before exercise

Yellow zone:
- Peak flow 170–270 (50 to 80 percent of personal best)
- Albuterol inhaler, two puffs four times a day
- Increase Pulmicort to two puffs twice a day for one week.
- Continue Uniphyl at one tablet in the morning. (Never increase the dose of theophylline without talking with your doctor; it's easy to overdose on it.)
- If not out of yellow zone in two to three days, see your doctor.

Red zone:
- Peak flow below 170 (below 50 percent of personal best)
- Start prednisone for a one- to five-day burst.
- Albuterol, four to six puffs every three to six hours
- Pulmicort, two puffs twice a day for one to two weeks
- Urgent (same day) visit with doctor
- Continue Uniphyl at one tablet in the morning.

Michael needed both a moderate dose of an inhaled corticosteroid and a long-acting symptom reliever. We chose the Pulmicort dry powder inhaler because it had less taste than other medicines and because it could be used once daily. We chose Uniphyl as his long-acting symptom reliever because he preferred a once-a-day pill to a twice-a-day inhaler.

After three weeks on this regimen, Michael started to notice a difference. He was hardly needing his albuterol and fully participating in physical education. He was sleeping better. He wasn't getting sick as much. And his teacher noticed that his attention in class was improved.

After six weeks, his best peak flow had improved to 360! We had to raise his green/yellow/red zone cutoffs to reflect his new personal best.

A Plan for Severe Asthma

Elizabeth is thirteen years old. She lives life with her lung function totally on the edge. One day, coming into the doctor's office during an asthma flare-up, she turned blue and passed out. Physical education and sports participation are out of the question. Emergency room visits and hospitalizations are regular events.

Elizabeth goes through two to three albuterol inhalers a month. Her peak flows bounce around a whole lot—she tends to be in the yellow zone much more than the green zone. She seldom wheezes, even though her peak flow readings are precariously low.

She misses a lot of school because of her illness, and her grades reflect it. She has already been left back twice. Her mom had to quit work just to be available to take care of her, and rush her to the emergency room whenever she needed it.

Getting Elizabeth's asthma into control is a challenge, but working together, we built a team that could tackle it. The team includes Elizabeth, her parents, an asthma nurse specialist and myself.

Elizabeth's mom quit smoking (with the help of a stop-smoking program). Allergy testing showed that Elizabeth was allergic to dust mites and to dogs, so we got allergen-proof encasings for her mattress and pillow. The dog got a doghouse outside. We diagnosed and treated Elizabeth's chronic sinus infection and her gastroesophageal (acid) reflux.

I felt that getting the inflammation of her breathing tubes beaten back was going to be tough. She was suffering. We needed quick results. I didn't feel that we could wait a month and a half (or more) for the maximal effect of her inhaled corticosteroid, so we started with a 14-day prednisone taper.

Why two weeks of prednisone? Prolonged courses of oral steroids are sometimes needed if the inflammation of the breathing tubes has been severe and long-standing. One note of caution: side effects are more common with a prolonged course of oral steroids. Expect some mood changes and weight gain.

If the oral steroid course has lasted longer than seven days, the dose must be tapered down gradually. The body needs some steroid in its system to function. After seven days, the adrenal gland's ability to make steroids may be suppressed. To get the adrenals working again, a steroid course needs to be gradually tapered off, with the dose decreased by only a little bit each day. Do not stop oral steroid medicine suddenly if they have been taken for more than seven days.

Elizabeth's Asthma Medication Plan

Personal best peak flow: 360

Green zone:
- Peak flow 300–360 (more than 83 percent of personal best)
- Flovent 220 micrograms per puff, two puffs, twice a day
- Serevent, two puffs twice a day
- Singulair, one tablet once a day
- Albuterol, two puffs before exercise

Yellow zone:
- Peak flow 200–300 (55 to 83 percent of personal best)
- Albuterol, two puffs four to six times a day
- Flovent, three puffs twice daily for one week only
- Continue Serevent at two puffs twice a day
- Continue Singulair at one tablet once a day
- If stuck in the yellow zone more than two days, a visit with a physician is needed.

Red zone:
- Peak flow below 200 (below 55 percent of personal best)
- Start prednisone for a one- to five-day burst.
- Albuterol, four to six puffs every three to six hours
- Flovent, three puffs twice a day for one week
- Continue Singulair, one tablet once a day
- See your doctor or go to the emergency room.

On this plan Elizabeth's lung function normalized. She was able—grudgingly—to resume participation in physical education. The hospital nurses started asking about her because they hadn't seen her for so long.

After two months of good control, we were able to back her Flovent 220 dose down to three puffs once a day.

ASTHMA ACTION PLAN

My Personal Best Peak Flow:_____
GREEN ZONE: Lungs are NORMAL. No Cough. No Wheeze. No Chest Tightness.

Peak Flow more than_____
❑ Take this medicine **EVERY DAY** to **PREVENT** asthma:
_____

❑ If there is cough, wheeze, or chest tightness when exercising take
_____15–30 minutes before exercise.
Other Medication:

YELLOW ZONE: Watch out. Starting to Lose Control.
Peak Flow_____to_____
❑ **Take** this medicine to **temporarily relieve asthma** symptoms:
_____

❑ **Increase preventive medication** for _____days.
_____

❑ Other Medicine:
Call your doctor or advice nurse if you are more than 2 days in yellow zone!

RED ZONE: AN ASTHMA FLARE-UP HAS STARTED. TAKE ACTION NOW!
Peak Flow under_____
❑ **To temporarily relieve asthma symptoms take:**
_____

❑ **To shrink the swelling** of the breathing tubes take:
_____

❑ **Increase preventive medicine** for _____**days.**
_____

❑ Other Medicine:
_____

Call your doctor or advice nurse! Your child needs to be seen!
Get medical care immediately if:
Very Fast or Hard Breathing
Sucking in the Stomach or Ribs to Breathe
Breathing so Hard You Can't Walk or Speak
Lips or Fingers Turn Blue
Best effort on Peak Flow is less than_____

PART III

Parents' Guide

10

Finding the Right Doctor

Of all the decisions you make about asthma, the first and most important is selecting the right physician.

Many people don't choose. They let their regular doctor treat their asthma. Or they see the specialist their family doctor recommends, or one they meet in the hospital.

Any of them may well be the best option. But it's worth making an *informed choice*, because the stakes are high.

There have been several studies finding that many patients do not receive care that follows basic National Institutes of Health (NIH) National Asthma Education and Prevention Program (NAEPP) asthma guidelines.[1] These guidelines, which underlie many of the elements of our program, have been proven to reduce hospitalizations, complications, and death. I believe that over the last several years, doctors—and patients—have improved; however, we still have a long way to go.

So why aren't the guidelines followed more often? I don't believe that it's because there are bad patients or bad doctors. But some powerful factors make it hard for physicians to keep up.

First, as we've seen, the field is changing fast. It's hard for doctors to keep up with all these advances, especially busy practitioners whose waiting rooms are full of every kind of medical problem imaginable.

Second, asthma requires a different approach from many other conditions.

In medical school, we learn that it's our job to prescribe the medicine and the patient's role to take it. Doctors are the experts—after all, that's why we have all those years of training. The patient really doesn't have to understand how the drugs work, and had better not change the way the medicine is taken without checking with the doctor.

Few of us, for example, were trained to let a patient change the dose of medicine, or start new powerful medicines on their own, at home. In many medical disciplines, that's a perfectly reasonable approach. For example, you wouldn't want a cancer patient adjusting his chemotherapy.

But asthma is different. The patient's situation changes season by season, day by day, minute by minute. Unless doctors are willing to follow patients around twenty-four hours a day, they must forge a different relationship—not as prescriber, but as consultant and educator—and leave the day-to-day management in the patient's and parents' hands. That's a big leap for many doctors.

Third, some doctors aren't aggressive enough when it comes to preventive therapy. This is one of the most common mistakes in asthma treatment.

The caution seems prudent—after all, asthma drugs are powerful, the lifestyle changes seem challenging, and the symptoms are often deceptively mild.

But the hard light of clinical research shows they're actually putting their patients at risk for more hospital stays, more crises, and even death. Undermedication increases the likelihood of crises, which in turn require higher doses of drugs.

Ironically, some doctors are also too cautious about *reducing* dosages after the asthma has been brought under control. Usually, once good asthma control is achieved you can maintain control with lower doses. Stepping down the dose of medication minimizes the chance of side effects. It really is a balancing act. Use enough medicine to maintain control, but not too much.

Fourth, some doctors don't take enough time. Especially at the beginning of the program, there's a fair amount of trial and error to see what works best for you. This requires the doctor's time and attention—

which are in short supply these days. It's also a reason why programs like ours use a nurse, respiratory therapist, or pharmacist as patient educators and patient advocates.

Rules for Finding a Good Asthma Doctor

So how do you find a good asthma doctor or improve the care you're getting from your current doctor?

At a minimum, a doctor who treats asthma should make sure that you and your child understand what the medications do, how to use them properly and what (if any) side effects to look for. He or she should also teach you how to prevent asthma, how to recognize flareups early and what to do about them if they happen; and should have a treatment plan aimed at *preventing* complications, not just managing them when they occur.

Beyond those general criteria, following are some practices you should look for:

1. A Good Doctor Gives You a Written Plan

If you're like me, if you don't write something down it probably doesn't get done. Most of us remember only a little bit of what we're told.

That's why Dr. Thomas Plaut, one of the pioneers of patient-centered asthma care, has a rule: *Good doctors give written instructions.*[2] A written self-management plan was key when he first wrote about it, and it is standard procedure now. The National Institutes of Health (NIH) recommends it and our own research shows how effective it is.[3]

The plan is not just any kind of instructions scribbled on the back of a sheet of paper. I hate to say it, but I've seen lots of badly written instructions. Some tell patients, "Do this now and come back if you have problems." Some are completely illegible. Others are too detailed, giving you so much information that you can't tell the forest from the trees. I saw one set, at a specialist's clinic in New Orleans, that went on for five pages. I couldn't figure it out. I can only imagine what patients went through—and how demoralized they must have felt.

Here are some criteria to consider for your asthma management plan:

* Is it legible?
* Is it simple?
* Is there anything I can't understand?
* Does it show my child and me how to monitor asthma?
* Does it tell us what to do when my child is feeling well?
* Does it tell us what to do when control is just starting to slip?
* Does it tell us what to do when there's a flare-up?
* Does it describe the medications my child is receiving and how to adjust them?
* Does it tell me when we need to see the doctor?
* Does it follow the green/yellow/red zone system recommended in the National Asthma Education and Prevention Program guidelines?

2. A Good Doctor Checks Technique

When asthma medications "don't work," it's often because they're not used correctly. With an inhaler, for example, the medicine you spray into your mouth doesn't do you any good; it has to get it into your lungs. It requires a certain breathing technique. A good doctor will watch how your child uses the inhaler or peak flow meter and offer suggestions on how to do it better. He or she will then periodically recheck and reinforce the technique.

3. A Good Doctor Will Figure Out Where You're Starting From

Asthma comes in many varieties. Some who have it barely know it's there. Others struggle with it constantly. The treatment plan starts with a good evaluation of whether your child's asthma is intermittent, mild, moderate, or severe.

This assessment is more than simply asking a few general questions about how you're feeling and how you think you're doing. It gets into specifics.

Many people underestimate their symptoms. I've had patients start by telling me, "I'm doing okay." But on further questioning, I find out that the patient is waking up a couple times a night with coughing. If I ask why she didn't tell me that in the first place, I often get an answer like, "Well, I use my inhaler and it's okay."

That's why it's important to get the details. Waking up twice a night is definitely not "doing okay." It tells me that the inflammation of the breathing tube is not being controlled and that the asthma is at a low smolder, waiting to flare up at any moment.

Here are some of the areas the doctor (or nurse) should ask about:

- How well your child is sleeping
- How he or she does with exercise
- How often he or she needs to use a symptom-relieving inhaler
- How long the inhalers last
- How often coughing, wheezing, or chest tightness occurs

5. A Good Doctor Will Check Your Child's Lung Function

Why measure lung function? Can't a good doctor evaluate asthma just by listening to the lungs?

Unfortunately, the answer is no. A person has to lose 25 percent or more of lung function before a skilled doctor will be able to notice something wrong by listening to the chest.

And patients vary. I have some patients who are exquisitely sensitive to what's going on in their chests. If it's the least bit tight, they feel it. But others are like Katelynn. She told me that she felt normal. I listened to her lungs and they sounded normal. But when I measured her lung function I got a big surprise. Her asthma was acting up more than she—or I—thought. If I hadn't made the measurements, I would have under-treated her.

6. A Good Doctor Is There
When There *Isn't* a Crisis

It's not enough for the doctor to be there when you need him or her. Her or she has to be there when things are going well, too. Prevention takes regular monitoring and assessment.

As busy as doctors are these days, not all of them see the need to spend this time with patients who "aren't sick."

There's no hard-and-fast rule about how often the doctor should see you and your child. It depends on the course of the disease and how well your plan is working. But by asking the question and listening closely to the answer, you can get a sense of whether the doctor views treatment as an ongoing preventive effort or simply management of occasional flare-ups.

7. A Good Doctor Is a Partner

Remember Maricella and her parents and their sense of hopelessness when I met them? When I see that sort of reaction, it often suggests that parents and patients haven't created a full partnership with their doctors.

Asthma treatment requires a different approach than, say, treating an ear infection or a broken arm. Because good asthma care involves behavior and lifestyle changes, treatment needs to be individualized and adapted.

The key to a good asthma plan isn't simply prescribing what *should* be done, but figuring out ways to be sure it *gets* done. You can't do that on your own. Your child can't. And neither can the doctor. It takes all of you working together.

For example, kids should use a peak flow meter to monitor their breathing, but sometimes they forget. Or think they don't have to. Or get embarrassed. So when they don't follow the rules, is it their fault? Or course not. They're kids. The key is to come up with new strategies that will work.

Your doctor knows the science and the techniques. You know your own circumstances. Together, you try things, make adjustments, and create a treatment plan that works for you.

8. A Good Doctor Shares Your Outlook

Beyond technical competence and qualifications lies a final—and per-haps the most important—consideration: whether there's a good "fit" between you and the doctor. That's hard to judge, especially at the outset.

One way to start is by first identifying your own goals for treatment.

They may seem obvious, but it's worth thinking them through and writing them down. Often, I've seen patients who feel at odds with their doctor without quite knowing why. When we probe a little deeper, it's usually because their goals aren't quite in synch.

For example, the doctor thinks Sally is doing just fine because her phys-ical symptoms are well controlled. But her parents are worried about her state of mind. Or the doctor recommends an increase in Daniel's dosage, but his parents would really rather try to control his environment more.

Often these conflicts lie just beneath the surface because parents and physicians haven't sat down and identified them. The doctor may be left with a vague notion that the parents aren't cooperative. The parents may conclude that the doctor isn't listening to them.

Here are some questions that can help you identify your goals. They don't have right or wrong answers; they're intended to provoke some thinking:

- How will *you* judge whether treatment is successful? How will your child?
- How do you feel about medication?
- What are the most difficult challenges you expect to face—for example, getting your child to take his medication, making lifestyle changes, dealing with the family and social issues?
- How does your child feel about her asthma?
- Describe what you expect your child's life to be like a year from now. How is it different from what it is today?

Another good way to get a sense of fit is by talking to other parents and children, using many of the same questions. Local support groups are a good place to start; you can find contact information in appen-dix C.

Specialist or Generalist?

You might think from all of this that I think asthma treatment should be left to the specialists.

Not so. I've known many pediatricians, internists, and family practice doctors who meet all of the criteria I've suggested, and, frankly, I've seen some specialists who don't. Knowledge, experience, and attitude are more important than credentials. In fact, our asthma program was built on the idea that the child's personal physician is the *best* choice for handling most cases of childhood asthma. They're the doctors who are most familiar with the patient, the entire family, and its history.

Our program didn't achieve its successes by sending lots of patients to specialists. Instead, we focused on helping front-line physicians gain the knowledge, skills, and tools they need to manage their patients' asthma.

You may need to see a specialist in some situations, but your first and best option is to work with your personal physician who understands what your child needs.

By the way, that doesn't necessarily mean changing doctors if you're not happy with the one you have (though on occasion it may). In our program, we've found that most doctors are open to new evidence and willing to try new approaches. Like most of us, they want to improve their skills. They want to give their patients the best possible care. And they want you to be satisfied.

That's why the role of patients and parents is so important. If you know what good asthma care looks like and expect to get it, you will. Chances are, you'll get it without having to change doctors.

Even when you do use a specialist, it's usually best to keep your family doctor involved as well, and to make both of them active partners with you. Depending on your situation, this partnership can take different forms. Sometimes your personal doctor can be the point person, helping you create a plan and coordinating the specialists' care. Sometimes the specialist takes the lead, working with parents to create a program and get it off the ground, and then bringing in your personal doctor for routine monitoring and follow-up.

.   .   .

When should you ask for a referral to a specialist? An asthma specialist is needed for severe or poorly controlled asthma. If, after working with your doctor for six months or more, your child is still waking at night due to coughing and wheezing, having difficulty with exercise, or needing repeated emergency room visits or hospitalizations, it's time to give someone else a try.

The National Asthma Education and Prevention Program guidelines say a specialist referral is needed when the patient:

- Has had a life-threatening episode of asthma
- Isn't meeting the goals of asthma therapy after three to six months of treatment (or earlier, if the doctor concludes that the patient isn't responding to treatment)
- Exhibits signs and symptoms that don't seem typical for asthma, or when there's a question about whether the diagnosis is accurate
- Needs additional education and guidance on complications of therapy or allergy avoidance, or has trouble adhering to the treatment plan

Who exactly is an asthma specialist? Most pediatric pulmonologists (childhood lung disease specialists), allergists (allergy specialists), and pulmonologists (adult lung disease specialists) include asthma as one of their areas of special expertise. A few pediatricians, internists, and family practice doctors may have a special interest in asthma and be able to take care of difficult asthma cases. Most good specialists will be board certified in their specialty. You can find out if a doctor is board certified by calling the American Board of Medical Specialties at 800-776-CERT.

Getting the Referral

Occasionally a doctor may be reluctant to refer to a specialist, or a health plan may be reluctant to pay for one.

If you believe your child needs a referral to a specialist, you can often get your health care provider on your side by actively advocating for what you and your child need. It may be an old saying, but it is true: The squeaky wheel gets the grease. If need be, you can cite the referral criteria from the National Asthma Education and Prevention Program (of the National Institutes of Health) guidelines given earlier in this chapter. Most doctors and most insurance companies want to provide good care for their patients and want satisfied customers.

11

Getting Your Health Plan On Board

Our experience at Vallejo and other Kaiser Permanente medical centers makes a convincing case that a comprehensive, prevention-oriented approach to asthma is not only good medicine but good business for health plans.

There's no question that poorly controlled asthma is expensive. More than half of the $7.5 billion annual health care costs for asthma is due to hospitalizations and emergency room visits.[1] Most of those can be prevented with good asthma management.

The first step is to have a regular doctor: a pediatrician for kids, an internist or family practitioner for adults. Research shows that good care from a regular pediatrician can go a long way toward improving asthma control.[2] Our research found that asthma control was much better for those who had a single doctor that they saw regularly.

Even "expensive" specialist care has been shown to have a positive impact on the bottom line for asthma care. Studies have shown that asthma specialists can reduce the need for the really expensive interventions like emergency room visits and hospitalizations.[3]

That doesn't mean everyone with asthma needs to see a specialist. As you've seen from examples in this book, many asthma patients who come to our center receive excellent care from their pediatrician. But when a child's asthma isn't in good control despite a generalist's best efforts, specialist care can save money by improving asthma control, preventing complications, and helping the patient avoid hospitalization.

I'm encouraged to see that more and more health plans have instituted some type of special program for asthma. Some, like us, follow the care manager model. Others take a different tack, for example, focusing on patient education. One innovative program in an inner city has focused on using community health workers—people from the community who have mastered their children's asthma and go on to help their neighbors.

Many such programs are relatively new, and it's too soon to tell which approaches will prove to be best. But in my view, all of them hold promise. I have to think that health plans that offer them are likely to be more enlightened about asthma care in other areas as well.

Choosing a Plan

You may or may not have the opportunity to choose a health plan. Some employers offer a number of options, but others give you only one. If you do have a choice, you can consider the criteria below. If you don't have a good plan, you can use this list to research other plans and bring them to the attention of your benefits manager when your company is renegotiating contracts. (It may help your cause if you can find coworkers who also have asthma or children with asthma.)

(NOTE: If you don't have a good health plan, check with local child welfare agencies. Your child may be eligible for various health programs or insurance, even if you don't qualify yourself.)

Health Plan Ratings

The National Center for Quality Assurance (NCQA) accredits managed care health plans. They produce a health plan report card. Plans are rated from no stars (worst) to four stars (best). Plans are rated in specific areas, including access and service—can you get an appointment when you need it; quality of qualified health care providers—how good are their doctors; staying healthy—preventive care services; getting better— treating illnesses; and living with illness—chronic care.

The NCQA is an independent, nonprofit organization whose mission is to evaluate and report on the quality of the nation's managed care organizations. Their ratings are so valuable that I would strongly suggest that you check them *before* you choose a health plan. You can easily obtain a health plan report card for the managed care plans in your area from their Internet site at http://www.ncqa.org.

What to Look For in a Health Plan

An enlightened health plan will:

- Have asthma education programs for asthma patients and their families
- Have special programs such as asthma case management to help with difficult-to-control asthma
- Seek out members with poorly controlled asthma to help get their asthma into good control (especially those with multiple emergency room visits and hospitalizations related to asthma)
- Have programs in place to bring the care given by generalists (pediatricians, family practitioners, and internists) up to the current standards as described in published NIH guidelines
- Provide access to allergy testing for patients with asthma
- Have stop-smoking programs available
- Provide access to good asthma specialists
- Work with schools and the community to improve asthma care resources
- Have an easy route to handle patient complaints
- Provide regular follow-up with their primary doctor or specialized nurse practitioner
- Promote asthma care guidelines that are consistent with NIH guidelines
- Have National Center for Quality Assurance (NCQA) accreditation if it is a managed care plan

A poor health plan will:

- Put up lots of barriers to obtaining asthma follow-up care
- Have little or no resources for asthma education

- Make it very difficult to see an asthma specialist
- Make no effort to ensure that the asthma care that its doctors deliver is current

Two key areas to consider are referral policies and pharmacy benefits. Some health plans put the doctors' personal income at risk every time they refer a patient to a specialist—the more they refer, the less money they make. Other health plans force a doctor to go through a complicated approval process *every* time he or she wants to refer someone to a specialist. In my view, these "cost-control" measures are penny-wise and pound-foolish, especially when it comes to asthma care.

The pharmacy benefit your plan offers can have a big impact on your pocketbook. Good asthma care requires preventive medications, quick-relief medications, devices to properly administer those medications (spacers, nebulizers) and devices to measure lung function (peak flow meters).

For some health plans, coverage only extends to medications. Devices such as spacers, nebulizers, and peak flow meters fall under the category of "durable medical equipment" (DME) and are covered only if you have DME coverage.

In addition, some health plans restrict you to generic medications. For most medications, generics are equivalent to brand name. However, it can get confusing when the medicine that you thought came in a blue inhaler now comes in a white or yellow one. I wish that we could convince the drug companies to standardize—one color for one medicine, no matter who makes it. Until then, it will be important for you to carefully look at the name of your medication and to know both its brand and generic name.

If You Don't Have Prescription Drug Coverage

If you don't have a pharmacy benefit, you can discuss with your doctor lower-cost alternatives. You can get a list of prices of similar medications from your pharmacist, and ask your doctor if less expensive medicines could be substituted. It pays to shop around if you have to pay for these medications out of pocket. The prices that pharmacies charge can be vastly different.

Many pharmaceutical companies have special programs for low-income persons without Medicaid coverage. You can ask your doctor to contact the company, or give a call yourself. You can find information about prescription drug assistance programs on the Internet at www. medicare.gov/Prescription/Home.asp.

If You Don't Have Durable Medical Equipment Coverage

If your child is hospitalized, some health plans will cover needed medical equipment as part of their discharge-planning process.

If you have to buy equipment, shop around. Some pharmacies or home care companies have large markups for equipment. The manufacturer sells it to the wholesaler, who sells it to the distributor, who sells it to the pharmacy, and each has tacked on a substantial markup. So sometimes you can save by purchasing direct from the manufacturer. I've seen a simple device like the AeroChamber, which Kaiser Permanente pharmacies are able to sell for about $11 (as we purchase in bulk direct from the manufacturer) sold by some community pharmacies for $40 and up!

Some allergy-supply houses will sell the devices through mail order at substantial discounts. Sometimes, if you spend a little more money than your insurance company authorizes, you can get a version that is easier to use, more attractive, or more convenient. If you can afford it, it's worth going for the equipment that you and your child will feel good about using every day.

Advocating with Your Health Plan

What should you do if you feel that you are not getting the coverage you deserve from your health plan?

The first and most basic principle: Ask. Physicians and most health plans want to keep their patients happy. It's surprising how much people get when they ask nicely. If your request is reasonable and is turned down, ask why. Ask what they would suggest as an alternative. If you're not happy with the response, ask to whom you could appeal the decision.

If you have to, take things up a step. For example, if you've been dealing with an advice nurse, ask to speak to a supervisor. Explain how your child's asthma has not been controlled, even after an adequate trial of medications as prescribed by your doctor, and that you would like to see a specialist. Or explain the severe complications of your child's asthma (multiple school absences, ER visits, hospitalizations, intensive care unit admissions, etc.) and explain that you feel this needs to be addressed by a specialist in asthma care.

If your child's primary physician is having trouble bringing the asthma under control but resists making a referral to a specialist, you may need to find another physician (see chapter 10). Sometimes, the level of care you get from your health plan has a lot more to do with your primary doctor's skill in negotiating the rules than with the plan itself.

If you must appeal, health plans have an appeals process to follow. Be sure to do your homework; a knowledgeable patient/parent is the best advocate. Review the appropriate sections of this book. Your "big stick" in an appeal is the National Institutes of Health expert panel report, which asthma experts agree forms the core of quality asthma care.[4] If you can show the care you're receiving doesn't meet these guidelines, I think most plans will be willing to give you what you need.

If all else fails, call the insurance commissioner's office in your state and ask for help.

Choosing and Using the Tools

In chapter 6 we discussed the principles behind the different devices used for medication delivery and for monitoring asthma. Here I want to give you more information about the different devices on the market, and how to choose and use the right one for your child.

As you recall from chapter 6, spacer devices (also called "holding chambers") help to get medication from a metered-dose inhaler into the lungs.

Spacer devices allow the larger particles contained in an aerosol spray to settle onto the walls of the spacer device. You don't want the large particles because they will not be able to make it to the small breathing tubes. If they didn't settle out in the spacer, the large particles would end up in your child's mouth and throat—where they can add to side effects without adding any beneficial effect.

The small particles are the ones we want. They can stay suspended in the center of the spacer device. They are the particles that can make it deep into the lungs. They are the particles that can benefit your child's asthma.

Spacer devices also decrease the need for coordination. Without a spacer, to use a metered-dose inhaler one must start breathing in a microsecond before puffing (actuating) the inhaler. This is hard enough for adults—forget about for a young child. With a spacer device, you puff, then breathe. It's much easier.

There are three different categories of spacer devices:

1. Tube type, also known as valved holding chambers (AeroChamber, AeroChamber with Mask, OptiChamber, EasiVENT, others)

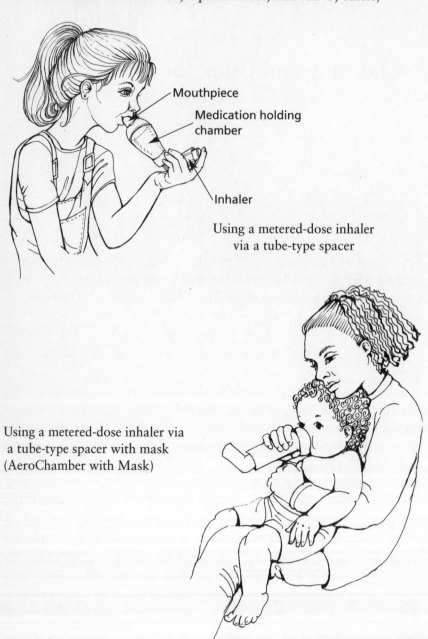

Mouthpiece

Medication holding chamber

Inhaler

Using a metered-dose inhaler via a tube-type spacer

Using a metered-dose inhaler via a tube-type spacer with mask (AeroChamber with Mask)

2. Bag-type holding chambers (InspirEase, EZ Spacer)

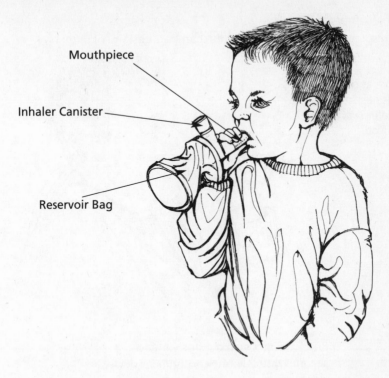

Mouthpiece

Inhaler Canister

Reservoir Bag

Using a metered-dose inhaler via a bag-type spacer

Tube-Type Spacers

A tube-type spacer is simply a small plastic tube. You insert the inhaler on one end. The other end has the mouthpiece (or mask) that you breathe the medicine in through. A series of one-way valves keeps the medicine going in the right direction.

The AeroChamber is the original and best researched of the tube-type spacers. Similar products include the OptiChamber and the EasiVENT.

The AeroChamber with Mask allows metered-dose inhalers to be used by infants and small children. I especially like the one-way valves. The valve to the medication chamber opens only when the child breathes in. An exhalation valve that bypasses the medication chamber opens when the child breathes out. So when the child exhales, the medicine doesn't blow out of the chamber. This one is the best mask delivery system I've seen.

3. Air-entrainment devices (OptiHaler)

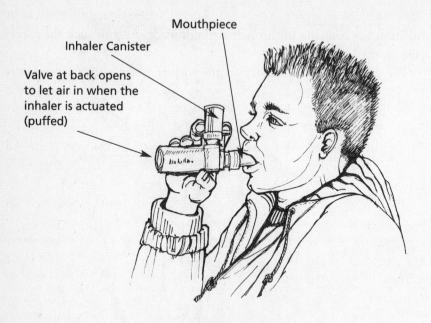

Mouthpiece

Inhaler Canister

Valve at back opens
to let air in when the
inhaler is actuated
(puffed)

Using a metered-dose inhaler
via an OptiHaler air-entrainment device

Tube-type spacers are easy to use and durable. They can be easily washed. It's possible for a child to break them, but it takes some effort.

Preschool and early school-age children tend to have difficulty with tube-type spacers. They're a little too old to use a mask, but when they use a mouthpiece their first instinct is to blow out, not to breathe in. It's difficult for them to grasp the idea that the medicine will enter their lungs if they breathe in.

Forgot to take the tube-type spacer to school? Not a problem. Take piece of 8½" × 11" paper. Roll it up into a tube. Place the inhaler in one end. Breathe in through the other. Though not "state of the art," it still functions as a perfectly adequate spacer.

Bag-Type Spacers

With bag-type spacers you spray the medicine into an inflated bag, then breathe the medicine in through a mouthpiece. As you suck the medicine in, the bag collapses.

The original bag-type spacer is the InspirEase. A copycat version is the EZ Spacer. With the InspirEase the bag goes out in front of the mouthpiece. With the EZ Spacer the bag goes down below the mouthpiece. For the InspirEase, the bag should probably be replaced monthly, the mouthpiece every six months. The EZ Spacer can be opened and cleaned. If you don't poke a hole in it, the EZ Spacer could last six months to one year.

The advantage of the bag-type devices is direct visual feedback. Kids don't have to imagine the medicine going in, as they do with tube-type spacers; they can see the bag inflating and deflating. This is a big advantage for the child in the four- to six-year age range. I have seen many a kindergartener who couldn't manage tube-type spacers but had no trouble learning to use an InspirEase.

The disadvantage of the bag-type spacers is that they don't last as long as the tube-type devices.

You can construct a simple bag-type spacer using the cardboard center of a toilet paper roll and a one-quart Ziploc bag. Cut one corner out of the bag, then insert the roll into it and tape it in securely. The roll serves as the mouthpiece. Place the inhaler inside the bag. Then seal the bag closed. Have your child blow through the tube to inflate the bag. Then have him or her spray the inhaler, filling the bag with mist, and inhale slowly through the cardboard mouthpiece.

Air-Entrainment Devices

Air-entrainment devices do the job of spacers, but in a slightly different way. They aren't holding chambers, so they do require coordination between spraying of the inhaler and breathing in. With the air-entrainment device, your child should spray the inhaler just as he starts to breathe in. The child should breathe in slowly and deeply, holding the breath for ten seconds, and then breathe out.

The device directs the medicine through a series of baffles, slowing down the medicine and filtering out the larger particles. Like the spacers, it increases the amount of medicine getting to the lungs while decreasing the amount that settles in the mouth.

The original air-entrainment device is the OptiHaler. The advantage of this device is its small size and stylish design. It fits easily in a small purse or pocket (making it popular with many teenagers). The disadvantage is that it requires coordination. You have to be able to spray and breathe in at the same time. Younger children have difficulty using this device.

Static Electricity

Static electricity on the walls of spacers can attract the small particles and so decrease the amount of medication that is available to your lungs. There's a simple way to remove this static electricity: Rinse the spacer in a diluted solution of dish detergent, then let it dry. The thin coating of detergent will prevent static electricity from accumulating, and increase the amount of medicine getting to your child's lungs.[1]

Choices in Nebulizers

Nebulizers are machines that take liquid medicine and make it into a mist for inhalation.

The different nebulizers on the market can be broken down into three categories:

1. Compressor-driven nebulizers
2. Portable, battery-powered nebulizers
3. Ultrasonic nebulizers

Compressor-driven nebulizers are the most inexpensive and the most common ones in use. I have seen some discount allergy suppliers selling models for under $100. The electric compressor blows a stream of air through tubing into a nebulizer cup, which holds the medicine. The stream of air is directed through the medicine and turns it into a fine mist. The mist then rises to the mouthpiece or mask.

Nebulizers with masks are best for infants and toddlers. Once children reach school age, most can breathe through a mouthpiece. If they can, the mouthpiece is preferable because less medicine is lost in the nose.

You have three choices of nebulizer cups to use with compressor-driven nebulizers:

- Disposable nebulizer cups (many brands). These devices need to be replaced at least monthly if they're in regular use.
- Dishwasher safe, reusable (Pari). The Pari nebulizer tends to be a little more efficient and a little faster than the traditional disposable nebulizer cups, making it a popular choice for home care. These nebulizer cups will last for six months to one year. The Pari Corporation makes a Pari Baby nebulizer, which has a mask that can swivel. That's a nice touch, because it lets you give a breathing treatment to a baby while she's lying down.
- Breath-actuated nebulizer (AeroEclipse BAN, Monaghan Medical Corp.). This is a new development in nebulizers. It creates a mist only when you breathe in. That leads to less medication waste. But be careful, especially if you're switching from another type. Because this type is more efficient than traditional models, the dose of medicine may need to be decreased.

Portable Nebulizers

These are nebulizers that work off a rechargeable battery. Some portable nebulizers have adapters that can be plugged into a car's cigarette lighter. Both ultrasonic and compressor-driven nebulizers are manufactured in battery-powered versions. As these devices are more expensive than conventional compressor-driven nebulizers, most insurance companies won't pay for them.

Ultrasonic Nebulizers

Ultrasonic nebulizers generate a rapid vibration that breaks the liquid up into a fine mist. Ultrasonic nebulizers are quiet and fast, but they're expensive. Many insurance companies won't cover the additional expense.

Choosing an Inhalation Device

Which inhalation device is the best? There's no one best solution for everyone; a lot depends on your child's age and preferences. But by and large, I lean toward the metered-dose inhalers. They're convenient, no mixing, no fuss, nothing to plug in, and they can be carried in a backpack, purse, or even a pocket. Nebulizers, by contrast, are expensive and require a power supply.

When used with a spacer device, a metered-dose inhaler can deliver medication to the lungs just as well as a nebulizer—and often in less time.[2] For example, about four to six puffs of albuterol given via a metered-dose inhaler with spacer (0.36 to 0.54 mg) have been estimated to give the same benefit as a nebulized breathing treatment with 2.5 mg of albuterol.

Whatever device you are using, correct inhalation technique is important. One of the most common reasons for poorly controlled asthma is poor inhaler technique. I have seen problems with every type of inhalation device. I've seen kids blow out instead of in through an inhaler. Or not remove the cap. Or fail to take a deep enough breath. With nebulizers, I've seen people put the mouthpiece in their mouth—and then proceed to breathe through their noses. I've seen parents hold the nebulizer mask away from the infant's face "so she can breathe." All of these examples underscore the fact that skill in use of an inhaler is not innate. It's not hard; it just needs to be learned—correctly. Be sure to have your doctor (or asthma nurse, or respiratory therapist) watch how you use your inhaled medicine.

HOW TO USE A METERED-DOSE INHALER WITH SPACER

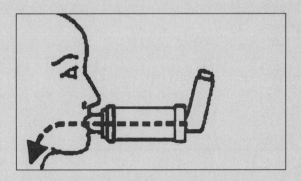

Using a metered-dose inhaler with spacer

* Remove the protective caps from the inhaler and spacer.
* Insert the inhaler into the spacer. (If using a bag-type spacer, be sure to untwist the reservoir bag gently to open it to its full size.)
* Place the mouthpiece of the spacer into your child's mouth. (For an infant, hold the AeroChamber with Mask tightly over the nose and mouth, making a seal.)
* Exhale (breathe out) normally.
* Actuate (spray) the inhaler so that one dose of medicine enters the spacer. For the air-entrainment devices (OptiHaler), start breathing in just before you actuate the inhaler. For tube (AeroChamber) or bag (InspirEase) spacers, start breathing in within a couple of seconds *after* you actuate the inhaler.
* Breathe in *slowly* and *deeply*. Fill the lungs completely. This full inspiration should take four to six seconds. Some devices will make a sound if the breath is too fast. (If using a bag-type spacer, like InspirEase, the bag should deflate completely.)
* Hold the medication within the lungs for 5 to 10 seconds before breathing out. (For an infant, allow 5 to 10 breaths while the

AeroChamber with Mask is held tightly over the nose and mouth. If the child is crying, it's okay; he is taking a deep breath and holding it.)

* Repeat until the full number of puffs that you and your doctor agreed on as part of your asthma self-management plan has been inhaled.
* When finished, be sure to replace the caps on the inhaler and spacer. (Imagine what would happen if a piece of something got in there and you didn't look before your child inhaled!)
* Be sure your child rinses and spits after using her inhaler. The medicine that ends up in her mouth is of no use to her.

HOW MANY PUFFS ARE LEFT IN A METERED-DOSE INHALER?

It can be difficult to tell when a metered-dose inhaler is empty because most inhalers will still spray even after the medicine is gone. The medicine dose is only reliable for the specified number of doses on the inhaler. Below are some strategies to use to tell when the inhaler is empty:

1. Divide the number of puffs used per day by the number of doses in the inhaler. For example, if there are 120 puffs in the inhaler and your child uses 2 puffs per day, then the inhaler will be empty after 60 days (divide 120 by 2). Write down the date 60 days from today on the inhaler. That is the day that you should consider the inhaler empty. (See table on page 80.)
2. Make a check on a piece of paper each time your child uses the inhaler. When the number of check marks equals the number of puffs in the inhaler, your inhaler is empty.
3. Use a counting device that advances by one number each time the inhaler is used. When the total number equals the number of puffs in the inhaler, it is empty.

4. Some inhalers can be floated in water. If it sinks it is full. If it floats horizontally on the top, it is empty. Note that the function of some inhalers (Intal, Nedocromil, QVAR, others) may be interfered with by placing them in water. *Always* check with your pharmacist before placing an inhaler in water.

HOW TO USE A TURBUHALER
DRY POWDER INHALER (FOR PULMICORT)

* Remove the cap.
* Hold the Turbuhaler with mouthpiece facing up when loading medicine.
* The first time the Turbuhaler is used it must be primed.
* To prime the unit, twist the brown grip to the right as far as it will go, then twist it all the way to the left until it clicks.
* Load a dose of medicine into the inhaler. Hold it upright, twist the brown grip to the right, then all the way to the left until it clicks.
* Breathe out normally. *Do not blow out into the inhaler*—you will blow out the dose of medicine. Do not shake the inhaler once a dose of medicine is loaded into it.
* Place the mouthpiece between your lips and teeth. Be sure to keep the Turbuhaler with mouthpiece pointing either up or horizontally.
* Breathe in through the Turbuhaler forcefully, rapidly, and deeply. Completely fill the lungs.
* Hold the breath for 5 to 10 seconds.
* Breathe out.
* Replace the protective cap and twist it shut.
* Always rinse the mouth with water after using inhaled corticosteroid medicine.
* Rinse and spit after using inhaled medication.
* Be sure to replace the cap after use.
* Keep the Turbuhaler dry. Store it in a dry location at room temperature.

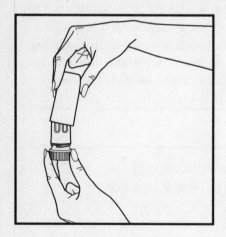

Removing the cover

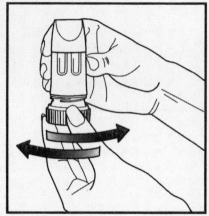

Loading the dose

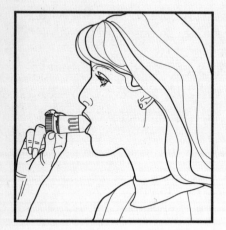

Breathing in the medicine

Using the Pulmicort Turbuhaler dry powder inhaler

HOW TO USE A NEBULIZER

- Measure the correct amount of medication into the nebulizer cup. Generally at least ½ tsp. (2½ ml) of medicine needs to be added to make an effective mist. If you need to dilute a concentrated medicine, use only "normal saline for inhalation." Do not use plain water.
- Fasten the mouthpiece or mask to the nebulizer cup.
- Turn on the air compressor machine. You should see a mist come out of the nebulizer.
- Place mouthpiece in mouth.
- Take slow, deep breaths. Breathe in through the mouthpiece (not through the nose).
- If using a mask, place the mask directly over the nose and mouth and breathe normally.
- Continue until the medicine is gone from the cup.

Measuring Lung Function: Peak Flow Meters

As you recall from the previous chapters, peak flow meters are simple devices that measure how forcefully a person can breathe out.

Home peak flow meters may not be completely accurate—you may use several different meters and get a slightly different result from each one. As we've seen, however, absolute accuracy isn't as important as consistency, that is, getting close to the same results every time you use it—assuming, of course, that lung function and effort have not changed.

Whichever meter you choose, always use the same one. Then you can compare measurements from test to test. If you use different meters, it's hard to know if the changes are due to your lung function or the differences in the meters.

Choosing a Peak Flow Meter

Many different types of peak flow meters are on the market. All do pretty much the same thing. The bells and whistles on each one are different. Here are some of the available options:

- Colored markers to indicate borders between green/yellow and yellow/red zones (available for most brands of peak flow meters)
- Attractive carrying case (Personal Best, HealthScan Corp.)
- Log scale: magnifies the lower range, compresses the upper range, so that one meter can be used for children, teenagers, and adults (TruZone, Monaghan Medical Corp.)
- Whistle: a meter set to whistle when you hit the green zone (Whistlewatch, Mallinckrodt Corp.)
- Asthma plan: a meter with space to write your green, yellow, and red zone plan on the back (AsthmaMentor, Respironics Corp.)
- Microprocessor: an electronic meter that displays your peak flow and lets you know if you are in the green, yellow, or red zone. It keeps a record of peak flows so that you can transmit them to your doctor over the phone lines (AirWatch). This fancy electronic toy is much more expensive than the other peak flow meters.

Some brands of peak flow meters offer "regular" and "low-range" models. The low range is nice for early-school-age children because they can blow the indicator farther up the meter. With a regular-range meter, their best possible effort would still have them at the bottom of the meter, which makes the results harder to read and can be demoralizing for the child. Generally, children under 50 inches tall and whose best peak flow is less than 250 liters per minute will do best with a low-range meter.

Log scale meters (TruZone) get around this problem by magnifying the lower ranges and compressing the upper ranges.

The most important thing in choosing a peak flow meter is in choosing one that will be used. A meter that will sit in a drawer will not do any good. If you think fancy bells and whistles will help your child to use it more reliably, go for it. If you or your child will enjoy using a fancier meter more, go for it. You will be using it every day for a long time to come, so you want to feel good about it. However, if expense is an issue, go for the cheapest one. It will give you the same information as the fancy, more expensive ones.

Peak flow meters can be purchased from most pharmacies and allergy supply houses (see listing in appendix C). Some of the manufacturers will also sell meters directly to consumers.

HOW TO USE YOUR PEAK FLOW METER

- Make sure the indicator is on zero.
- Fill your lungs with as much air as they will hold.
- Place the mouthpiece of the meter in your mouth.
- Blow out as hard and fast as you can.
- Repeat three times. Take the best of the three as your peak flow rate.
- Record your peak flow in your asthma diary.

13

Asthma through the Seasons

Consider this scenario: You've worked hard to get your child's asthma under control, and you and the doctor have come up with a plan that's working well. The flare-ups have subsided. Your child is breathing easier, sleeping better, and going to school every day.

Then, three months later, everything falls apart.

Does that mean you weren't on the right track? That the medications stopped working? That your child built up tolerance to them?

Probably not.

Chances are, the seasons changed. And when the seasons change, the rules for asthma treatment often change along with them. A control strategy that worked fine in the summer may completely fall apart when cold weather sets in.

The asthma triggers that your child encounters may change with the seasons. If tree and grass pollen is a big factor, then spring and summer may be your child's worst seasons. If viral infections (like colds) are your child's big trigger, then winters may be worst.

To get the greatest control with the least medication, you may need to adjust your plan for the season, increasing medication in your child's worst season(s), decreasing medication for his or her best season(s).

Once we doctors point out the seasonal nature of asthma to parents and kids, we can almost see the light going on over their heads. Usually the patterns are clear once we look for them. "Of course," Mom realizes. "Janie always gets a bad cold in the first couple of weeks of school." That's a powerful piece of knowledge as you tackle your child's asthma in the future. Maybe Janie needs preventive medicine (like inhaled corticosteroid) restarted or increased, starting a couple of weeks before school. It won't keep her from getting the cold, but it may make it less likely to trigger her asthma.

I have some patients whose asthma flares up every year like clockwork right around the holidays. Is it the stress and strain of the season? Maybe. But a more likely explanation is that the beautiful Christmas tree is throwing off volatile oils that are irritating the lungs.

Once patients begin to sense the seasonal rhythms of asthma, they gain a greater sense of control. They begin to see a certain logic to the disease. They see that flare-ups usually happen for a reason, and don't just strike out of the blue. So parents and kids feel less blindsided by this disease, and see how they can stay a step ahead of these seasonal changes.

Winter

For many people with asthma, winter is the worst season. They're spending more time indoors. Colds and flu are in the air. Fireplaces are roaring—and throwing out smoke and soot. All those boughs of holly decking the halls, not to mention the pine and spruce, are oozing asthma triggers.

If winter is your child's worst season, you may need to increase preventive medicines during this time. Pay more attention to peak flow and to asthma symptoms, knowing that the risk for problems is a little higher.

Of course, you need to discuss this strategy with your child's doctor before you make any changes; you don't want to be giving your child more medicine than necessary. It's helpful to look at past experience: How was your child's asthma in prior winters?

In addition to adjusting the medication plan, it pays to look at specific triggers and take preventive measures. One of the most significant is colds and viruses. The best way to avoid colds is just what your mother taught you as a young child: Wash your hands. Often. Hand washing has a "dose-response" effect: The more often you wash, the fewer colds you'll get.

Colds are spread when you pick up the virus from touching someone else or a contaminated surface, and then touch your nose, eyes, or mouth. Hand washing breaks this chain of infection.

Other viruses pose a greater challenge. I had one patient, a sweet teenage girl whose asthma had always been mild, yet when I met her, she was in the intensive care unit, fighting for her every breath. Lab tests showed she was infected with influenza.

After we helped her through this episode and her flu cleared up, we were able to get her asthma back under control. Now she gets her flu shot every year, and she's been doing well ever since.

The moral? For kids with asthma, flu shots are one of the simplest things you can do to head off a flare-up.

It's a good idea to eliminate or reduce other winter triggers. Go ahead and put logs in the fireplace. Just don't light them. Get an artificial Christmas tree. And don't forget your heating system. If you have forced-air heating, make sure the filters are fresh and clean. If possible, get high-efficiency filters to cut down on the amount of dust that gets recirculated.

The cold dry air in the winter can sometimes bring out trouble. Wearing a scarf or mask over the nose and mouth can help to warm and humidify the air.

Spring

If your child is allergic to pollen, spring will likely be the toughest asthma season. Pay careful attention to peak flow readings to detect flare-ups early and, if necessary, increase preventive medicines. If you know from past experience that once everything starts to bloom your child will be having asthma problems, talk to your doctor about starting or increasing preventive medicines for the allergy season. Remember to take the medicine dose down again once allergy season is over.

Don't forget about the nose. Allergy symptoms in the nose sometimes are connected to asthma symptoms in the lungs. If hay fever (allergic runny, itchy nose) is a problem, consider using an antihistamine or other anti-allergy medicine, such as cromolyn nose spray (Nasalcrom) or a corticosteroid nose spray (Beconase, Rhinocort, Flonase).

Summer

If viruses and indoor allergens are the major problems for your child, summer may be your child's best season. If so, talk to your doctor about cutting back on preventive medicines for the summer.

How will you know if your child can use less medication? Follow peak flow rates. If peak flows are rock-solid stable in the green zone and there are no asthma symptoms, talk to your doctor about tapering off on the medicine doses. If the peak flow stays solidly in the green zone and your child remains symptom-free for the next several weeks, things are fine. But if the peak flow starts to bounce around and asthma symptoms begin to appear, go back to what you were doing before. *Always* discuss medication changes with your doctor.

On the other hand, if your child is allergic to grass and outdoor molds, asthma may worsen in the summer. You may need to *increase* preventive medication.

Keep in mind that each geographic area has its own seasons for the different allergens. In California, the grasses go crazy in the spring, then often die out for the dry summer. In the Northeast, ragweed finds the late summer a wonderful time to pollinate. Allergy testing can help you identify what your child is allergic to (see pages 46–47). Then pollen counts can help you identify what is out there and when—so you can be prepared. You can find the pollen and mold spore counts in your area from the National Allergy Bureau. Call 800-9-POLLEN or use their Web site, http://www.aaaai.org/nab/pollen.stm.

Be sure to keep the air-conditioning filters fresh and clean. Air conditioning can be a big benefit for kids with asthma; it helps to keep the humidity down—and hence mold growth—and the filter helps keep pollen, dust, and other triggers out of the air.

Evaporative coolers—also known as "swamp coolers," commonly used in hot dry climates—aren't good for asthma. Their moisture tends to attract lots of mold. Regular air conditioning is better.

Fall

One of the big challenges in fall is when kids come back to school and start trading summer stories—and respiratory infections. You may need to restart or increase preventive medications, especially if they were reduced for the summer.

On the other hand, for some children fall and winter are the good seasons. If this describes your child, talk to your doctor about stepping down the medication for the fall and winter.

Prepare for the coming winter. October is a great time for everyone in the family to get a flu shot. An annual influenza vaccination is important for both adults and children with asthma. Just about any child over six months old can get a flu shot.

14

Infants and Toddlers

Infants and toddlers with asthma are a special challenge. They won't inhale when you tell them. They won't blow out when you tell them. And flare-ups can worsen rapidly. What do you do?

Though they can't do a peak flow maneuver, infants and toddlers can tell you what they feel. It may not be with a word, but instead with a cry or a look. It may be their pattern of activity, a change in their appetite, a change in sleep habits, or a change in their breathing.

Though they can't take a deep breath on command, by using devices like the AeroChamber with Mask or a nebulizer you can give inhaled medicine to a baby.

Is It Really Asthma?

I have had many a parent come to me angry with their regular doctor. They say that their infant has had a couple of wheezing episodes—episodes that sounded just like asthma. The doctor wouldn't call it asthma, but instead said it was reactive airways disease. Or bronchiolitis. Or wheezing associated with respiratory illness, or a wheezy cold—anything but asthma. Why?

In the late 1980s I was taught that you don't diagnose asthma until a child is two years old. Furthermore, we didn't want to "label" a child as having asthma to avoid the "stigma," which might cause them difficulty in getting health insurance.

But in the early 1990s, spurred on by parent advocacy groups such as Mothers of Asthmatics, we began to rethink these attitudes and realized we weren't saving parents any grief by delaying the diagnosis. Once we identified asthma, a whole range of preventive and treatment opportunities opened up. Parents felt empowered. They knew what to expect. They could make plans. And they didn't have to live in fear of what might be going on from illness to illness.

But by the late 1990s, we were also starting to understand that different processes could cause wheezing in infants. Sometimes it *would* be just a bad cold. Other times it would be asthma. Frequently it was both.

A study from Tucson, Arizona, found that about a third of infants had a wheezing illness. But by the time they were six years old, more than half of them no longer wheezed.[1] They seemed to grow out of it.

Two factors seemed to help in predicting which babies would continue wheezing: a family history of asthma and exposure to cigarette smoke. This information helps us make an educated guess about which babies will grow out of it, but it doesn't allow us to predict a child's future with anything close to 100 percent certainty.

So what advice can be given to a parent whose baby has a wheezy cold? To give this child the best chance for maximum lung function, a smoke-free environment is critical. That is one thing we can change.

We can't change our genes (at least not yet). If you yourself have a history of asthma, and your baby has wheezed, there's a good chance that your baby will go on to have asthma. On the other hand, if there's no one who had asthma or allergies in your family and no one smokes, then there's a pretty good chance that the baby will grow out of it.

Though we can make a guess about how a baby will do based on family history of allergies and asthma, it is difficult to tell for sure until the baby has gotten old enough to develop a track record. Yet even this indicator isn't 100 percent reliable. I have seen many a baby who had very difficult times as an infant go on to have much milder problems as they got older. I've also seen it go the other way.

All that notwithstanding, waiting to grow out of asthma is no way to manage it. The children are suffering now. Furthermore, the evidence suggests that for children with chronic, persistent asthma symptoms (and therefore chronic inflammation of the breathing tubes), the earlier in life we get the asthma—and the inflammation—into control, the milder their asthma may be as they get older.[2]

A Practical Approach

By and large the basic principles of treatment are the same for infants as for everyone else. We need to assess the asthma: Is it intermittent and mild, or are symptoms persistent or severe? Are asthma triggers (especially smoke) removed from the home environment?

If asthma is intermittent and mild, a quick-acting symptom reliever used occasionally may be sufficient treatment. If it's persistent or severe, then it's important to use preventive medicine every day. This reduces the inflammation that causes asthma. Follow up with your doctor to find the lowest dose of medication that will keep the asthma well controlled.

If asthma is not well controlled, see your doctor. Often, consultation with a pediatric pulmonary specialist is needed. Sometimes the coughing and wheezing isn't caused by asthma, but by something else entirely.[3]

Quick Relievers

The most commonly used quick-relief medicine for infants is albuterol (Proventil, Ventolin).

This medication can be taken by mouth (as a syrup) or inhaled using either an AeroChamber with Mask or a nebulizer. When choosing which route to give the medicine (swallowed or inhaled), you want to balance the need for ease and convenience against the need for effectiveness. Of course, always be sure to discuss asthma medication plans with your doctor. The detailed information on medication given below will help you to have a more informed discussion with your doctor.

Oral Medicine

Giving a teaspoon of a sweet syrup by mouth is often much easier and quicker than to try to get a child to sit still for a breathing treatment.

However, because the oral route gets less of the medication to the lungs, it's less effective.

Nebulized Medicine

Giving a breathing treatment by nebulizer gets a higher dose of medication to the lungs, but you need an expensive machine, a power supply, and need to get the child to sit still for ten to fifteen minutes or so.

Inhaler with Spacer

A metered-dose inhaler with spacer (AeroChamber with Mask) can be just as effective as a nebulizer, if enough puffs are used. This approach has the convenience of portability. The challenge is getting the child to put up with having a mask held snugly over his face. (See the lower illustration on page 140.)

Long-Acting Preventive Medications

For the long-acting (preventive) asthma controllers, oral medicine for babies is not an option. Your choices are restricted to cromolyn (Intal) and the inhaled corticosteroids, delivered either by a metered-dose inhaler or a nebulizer.

Due to its excellent track record of safety, your doctor may want to try cromolyn first, especially if asthma is relatively mild. If the cromolyn doesn't seem to be working by the end of the first month, try a low dose of an inhaled corticosteroid.

If the infant has moderate persistent asthma, you may need to go directly to a low to medium dose of an inhaled corticosteroid. If a medium to high dose of inhaled corticosteroids is needed for a baby, consultation with a pediatric asthma specialist is warranted.

Cromolyn

How should cromolyn be administered? In the United States, the nebulized preparation contains twenty five times more medicine than a puff on the cromolyn inhaler. For this reason, I prefer to give cromolyn via a nebulizer machine. For maximum effectiveness, it needs to be given at least three to four times per day.

Inhaled Corticosteroids

For moderate to severe asthma, inhaled corticosteroids are the most effective asthma controller medication available. Low-dose inhaled corticosteroid medication has an excellent track record of safety.

Inhaled corticosteroids are available in the United States as a metered-dose inhaler medication. A nebulizable preparation of the inhaled corticosteroid budesonide (Pulmicort Respules) has recently become available in the United States.

Should we all jump on the bandwagon of nebulized budesonide? My feeling is not to jump too high nor too soon. Nebulizing a corticosteroid medicine has several disadvantages. Dosing is unreliable, much of the medicine goes into the surrounding environment (to be breathed in by others in the room), and some of the medicine may deposit in the eyes, which may increase the risk for cataracts. On the other hand, if a young child has severe, difficult-to-control asthma and lots of trouble using a metered-dose inhaler via AeroChamber with Mask, nebulized budesonide might be useful.

There are some downsides of using inhaled corticosteroids for infants. A small decrease in growth rate may be seen (see chapter 7), though the effect on final height is probably minimal. At low doses, this is rarely a problem, but make sure that your doctor carefully monitors your baby's growth if inhaled corticosteroid medications are used.

The other downside is that for babies with small lungs, most wheezing is caused by viruses (like the viruses that cause the common cold). Viral-induced inflammation is difficult to stop completely. However, a concerted effort at asthma control can at least blunt some of the damage. Careful attention to handwashing can help prevent viral infections.

Asthma Management Plans for Infants

For babies, we use the same principles of green/yellow/red zone management that were discussed in chapter 9.

Since infants can't use a peak flow meter, you have to look at both asthma symptoms and breathing rate to tell whether they're in the green, yellow, or red zone.

If there's no coughing or wheezing and breathing rate is normal, they're in the green zone.

If there is an occasional mild cough or wheeze they are in the yellow zone.

If there is rapid breathing, persistent coughing or wheezing, with so much difficulty breathing that they have trouble sleeping or eating, sucking in the chest or abdomen with each breath, flaring of the nostrils with each breath, or working hard to breathe, they're in the red zone. You don't have to have all of these findings to be in the red zone. Any one of them alone would make me concerned.

A breathing rate (at rest) from 20 to 40 breaths per minute is normal for an infant. A breathing rate from 18 to 30 breaths per minute is normal for a toddler. Count and record your baby's breathing rate on a regular basis so that you get used to her normal breathing pattern.

For the green zone, control asthma triggers in the home, especially smoke and strong chemicals. If the child is well between asthma flare-ups, and the flare-ups are infrequent and mild, then no medicine is needed in the green zone. If the child has frequent coughing and wheezing (more than one week a month) then talk to your doctor about daily use of a long-acting asthma controller (cromolyn or an inhaled corticosteroid) to keep asthma in control.

For the yellow zone, talk to your doctor about adding on a quick-relief medication. If you're using an inhaled corticosteroid, ask the doctor about increasing the dosage for one to two weeks.

For the red zone, your doctor may add a short "burst" of an oral corticosteroid (such as prednisolone) in addition to your quick-relief medication. In the red zone your child needs medical attention. Call or visit your doctor. If your doctor isn't available, bring your infant to an emergency room.

15

Teenagers and Asthma

The teenage years are difficult ones, especially for kids with a chronic illness. A condition like asthma seems to touch on the classic issues of adolescence: the desire to fit in, the desire to test limits, the need to be independent.

Even if kids were agreeable about taking medicine every day when they were younger, their attitudes may change for the worse when they reach the teenage years. All of a sudden they'll have a million reasons why they don't "need" to take their medications. Or, worse, will tell you they're taking them when they aren't. A lot of these attitudes are related to asserting their independence.

For many teens, smoking becomes a big issue. Sometimes there is the peer pressure to smoke. Sometimes the parents modeled it. Even if your teen doesn't smoke, he or she may be around others who do. Of course it's illegal for teens to smoke. But in the real world, that just makes it more appealing.

What's a parent to do if her teenager has asthma? First, try not to make too much of a fuss. Let your child know that having asthma is not a big deal, and that lots of their classmates, friends, sports stars, and many celebrities have asthma.

Also, try to avoid saying, "My child can't *(fill in the blank)* because of asthma." Focus on what they *can* do, which for most teens with asthma is just about anything except smoking.

Reinforce the need to take asthma medicine, and the reasons why. But try to stay matter-of-fact about it. If you make a big deal over it, your teenagers may try to turn it into a battle over parental control and their independence. Let them challenge you on something else.

Role models are important for teens. Kids pick up many more of their parents' habits than we like to admit—both their good habits and their bad ones. If a parent neglects his or her own asthma (or other chronic illness), the child will feel that he or she can ignore theirs too.

Transfer responsibility for taking medication to the child, in an age-appropriate manner. Hanging on to control leads to struggle and conflict. Teenagers need to take ownership of their asthma care.

Yet the teenager still needs to know that his or her parent cares. They want responsibility, but may not have the skills to fully handle it. Find ways to check up on your teen without being intrusive. If a medication canister stays in the same position in the same place for days on end, it is probably not being used. Trust, but verify.

It's often useful for teens to get some time with their physician by themselves. This helps them feel they're in charge of their own care, and it allows them to bring up *their* concerns. When a parent is in the room, the parent often dominates the conversation. The parent is used to reporting on the child's health. The doctor may find the parent easier to relate to. Give your teen some time alone with his or her doctor.

Medications are a big issue. I find that it's important with teenagers to ease the burden of asthma treatment as much as possible. The simpler the regimen, the more likely it is to be followed. Once-daily medications are better than those that need to be taken several times a day. In the same way, two puffs will work better than four or six.

Spacers are another issue. Suddenly, kids who've used them for years decide they're "dorky" or "lame." Size matters: Large bulky tubes or bags that don't fit in pockets are likely to be left home or in the school bag. Attractiveness matters, too. If a teenager must be seen with a spacer, it had better be a good-looking one.

I've found many teens prefer a dry powder inhaler for their corticosteroids because it's smaller and doesn't need a spacer. Others who don't like an AeroChamber or other tube-type spacer will use a smaller air-entrainment device such as the OptiHaler.

If there's a lot of conflict between a parent and a teen about self-care for asthma, the issues may be deeper than just asthma. The conflict may reflect depression, anger, hopelessness, difficulty adjusting to life with a chronic illness, or just a struggle for control. In these situations, family therapy is often very beneficial for both the parents and the child.

16

Asthma outside the Home

The steps you take at home will go a long way toward helping your child take control of asthma. But eventually they have to leave the nest.

Out in the rest of the world, the rules are different. Whether you're dealing with schools, visits to the homes of friends and family, or just a trip to the mall, you can't exert the same degree of direct control as at home.

To a certain extent, it will be up to you, but ultimately it will be up to your child to manage in these environments and situations. When he must be in less-than-ideal environments, he has to be aware of how his lungs are responding and, if needed, use appropriate medications to head off flare-ups.

Other skills are equally important, such as a willingness to speak up. Parents and kids need to learn how to advocate, educate, persuade, and, at times, insist on what they need to protect their health.

Schools

Besides your home, the place your child spends most of her time is in school.

Schools present two kinds of problems for kids with asthma:

1. The facility itself. Many schools are full of asthma triggers: chalk-boards, molds, dust, viruses, small furry animals in the back of the class, poorly ventilated chemistry labs, poorly maintained ventilation systems. I have even seen some schools cut the grass right when the kids who are allergic to it are on it. Some schools are better than others, but any place that's full of kids and activities may have asthma triggers.

2. Attitudes. These can be even more challenging than the physical facility. Teachers, administrators, support staff, even the school nurse (assuming there is one) may not understand what your child needs to keep her asthma in control. You could probably add your own stories to the ones that I hear every day. "School policy won't let my child carry his inhaler." "The teacher told my child to wait until the end of the period to go to the office for her breathing treatment." Then there's the gym teacher who insists that your child run even when asthma is start-ing to flare up, support staff who feel unqualified and resent being put in charge of the child's medication, or school administrators who may refuse to take even the simplest steps to reduce asthma triggers.

But from another perspective, these attitudes can represent an oppor-tunity for parents. You can educate school personnel about what kids with asthma need. You can advocate for changes. And because asthma is so common, you can probably team up with other parents who are facing the same challenges.

Many teachers and administrators are afraid of asthma. Their train-ing is teaching students—not providing health care. They're afraid of adverse effects of medication, afraid the child will not be responsible with medication, and afraid the child might "abuse" the medicine, give their inhaler to another child to use.

What's more, many school districts have gotten away from the idea of a nurse at every school. Often the school secretary is in charge of handling and administering medications. Many do a good job, but many others feel, quite rightly, that this is a responsibility they weren't trained for.

Some teachers, support staff, and administrators may well have some very different beliefs about asthma than you or your physician. For example, they may think "less is more" when it comes to medica-tions, and discourage kids from asking for or using their inhalers. They don't even have to say anything to send that message—a sigh or a disapproving look may be all it takes for kids to feel they're doing something wrong.

Teachers may have difficulty telling when an asthma flare-up is real or faked. They are concerned about children "using" their asthma to get out of things. They are concerned about children using their asthma to "manipulate" them. In other cases, the pendulum may swing the other way—they may want to restrict a child with asthma from full participation in activities when there's no need to do so.

What Schools Need to Know

Parents, in teamwork with their doctors, can take the lead in educating teachers and others about asthma symptoms.

Several of my more ambitious parents have given seminars to school personnel about asthma. At Kaiser Permanente in Vallejo, we produced an award-winning video to help educate school personnel about asthma, called *Taming Asthma*. The National Heart Lung and Blood Institute (NHLBI) also has asthma information for the schools.

Here are the key issues school personnel should know about asthma:

- How to recognize asthma symptoms
- What to do if asthma flares up
- How to know when asthma is not in good control and when to alert the school nurse, parents, or the child's doctor.
- Special needs of kids with asthma. They may need to take medicine before physical education classes, or they may need to rest and take quick-relief medicine if asthma symptoms develop or peak flows decrease. They may need to cut back on activity if asthma is in the yellow zone.

But we adults also need to do our part. School nurses tell me that some parents don't even tell them that a child has asthma. Or they discover on the day Joey has an asthma attack that the quick-relief inhaler was left at home. Or they can't get a copy of his written asthma management (green/yellow/red zone) plan.

I believe that most schools want to do the right thing for children with asthma. We need to be sure to give them the tools to enable them to do so.

I've included a sample letter at the end of this chapter that you can adapt to give basic instructions to your child's school. In addition to the letter, be sure to give the school a copy of your child's asthma management green/yellow/red zone plan. Go over the plan with the teacher and whoever is responsible for handling medications at the school. Make sure you give the school a peak flow meter, so they can check your child's lung function and find out how bad the asthma is. And always keep an extra quick-relief inhaler at school.

Asthma in the Curriculum

As more and more school-age children are diagnosed with asthma, many schools are looking at adding the subject to the curriculum. It's a rich topic, ranging from the science of why asthma occurs to the interpersonal issues related to kids feeling "different" from their peers. In my experience, when the whole class learns about asthma, it makes life better for everyone. Usually, the other kids take it in stride—in fact, they often start to help their classmates with asthma stick with their program. The biggest benefit is that they just become more comfortable with the idea that one or more of their classmates has asthma. And that takes some of the stress off teachers and others as well.

The American Lung Association has designed an education curriculum for elementary school children called "Open Airways." Another asthma education curriculum is available from the National Heart Lung and Blood Institute, "Asthma Awareness." The Asthma and Allergy Foundation of America has an excellent asthma education curriculum for teenagers, "Power Breathing."

On a related note, many American Lung Association chapters run asthma camps in the summers. They're a great way for kids with asthma to learn about what they need to do to keep their asthma in control and to meet other kids who face the same challenges.

Asthma Triggers in the Schools

Schools can be an important source of asthma triggers. Sometimes the reason for difficulty in controlling asthma lies at school.

I had a patient who had a most difficult time getting her asthma into control. We couldn't figure out why—until we found out about the rabbit in her classroom! Her parents hadn't wanted to make an issue of it—depriving other children of their rabbit wouldn't be fair and might cause some resentment. But when we saw what a big impact it had on the child's breathing, they decided to discuss it with the teacher.

The teacher was completely sympathetic. She found another home for Bunny, and the child's breathing improved and her need for medication decreased. Everyone at school felt good because of the simple help that they were able to provide for her—help that made such a big difference in her life.

I can't say these stories always have such happy endings. And I can understand parents' reluctance to rock the boat. But in these kinds of situations, teachers and other students are often willing to be accommodating. In fact, enlightened teachers often use these kinds of issues as "teachable moments," that is, an opportunity to deliver a real-world lesson about tolerance and accommodation.

I had another patient, Ronny, who had severe mold allergies. We had a tough time bringing his asthma into control until we found that there was a leak in the roof at his school. The ceiling was growing lots of mold and mildew. In this case, *I* contacted the school and explained the problem; we thought we'd get a quicker response if the school heard from a physician rather than a parent. It worked. The school fixed the roof and removed the mold from the ceiling. Ronny has done much better since then.

Other issues may be more difficult to deal with. Though many schools are officially smoke-free, lots of times high school kids are still sneaking smokes in the bathroom. With smoking banned in the buildings, many times smokers crowd around outside the entrances, forcing anyone entering or leaving to run a gauntlet of dense smoke. I'm optimistic that this will change someday as more and more people give up smoking altogether.

Friends and Family

Sometimes, however, the public spaces are easier to deal with than those of our friends and family. How can you tell someone not to smoke in his or her own house? Are you going to decide not to visit friends or family just because they smoke? And of course simply asking them to refrain from smoking while your child is visiting won't do much good if the home is already filled with smoke. Maybe the solution is to have them over to your home instead—then it's much easier to ask them to step outside for their cigarette.

In our practice, I hear over and over again from parents frustrated by family-and-friend issues. They always hit deep emotional hot buttons—parents' relationships with their own parents, issues of autonomy and control, respect issues. Some grandparents think the parents are over-protective. Some think they're not careful enough. Friends may feel offended, their lifestyles judged.

There's no simple prescription. About the best advice I can offer is to practice patience and persistence. Parents tell me they're more successful when they can keep the discussion focused on asthma and the role of triggers, instead of on interpersonal issues and emotional baggage. It boils down to a simple proposition: We know that certain things in the environment trigger asthma attacks. We can keep kids healthier by reducing their exposure to those triggers. That's really the only thing at issue.

Friends and family don't come around all at once (neither, for that matter, do parents and patients). It takes time for people to learn, understand, and ultimately accept these ideas. Frankly, some people never do, but eventually, I find, most do work out some sort of accommodation that protects their kids' health and their relationships with family and friends.

Asthma Triggers in the Community

You hear a lot about air pollution and other contaminants contributing to asthma. There is no question that pollution from large smokestacks and factories can trigger asthma. But bigger problems often lie closer to home.

A couple of the biggest problems come from two common asthma triggers: tobacco smoke in public places and automobile exhaust.

Though some states and cities restrict smoking in public buildings, others do not. "Nonsmoking" areas of a restaurant are a joke if they share the air with a smoking area. A smoking area in a mall will affect everyone in the mall unless it has a completely separate air circulation.

Automobile (and diesel) exhaust generates especially small particulate matter. So the small particles in automobile exhaust stay suspended in the air and can easily get down deep into your child's lungs, where they can trigger asthma.

Children with asthma may need to stay indoors, in an air-conditioned environment, when air-pollution levels are high.

The Big Picture

I believe that those of us involved with or affected by asthma—doctors, nurses, educators, and parents—have a special responsibility to speak out for a cleaner environment.

Clear associations between air pollution and asthma have been demonstrated. For example, in rural Louisiana, you could expect asthma to start flaring up when they started to burn the sugar cane. Both New Orleans and Barcelona, Spain, have reported "epidemics" of asthma associated with unloading of soybeans from ships, which spread allergens through the neighboring community.[1] In California, we have lots of people who like to use fireplaces and wood-burning stoves. You can try as you might to keep your home smoke-free, but when you go outside, you find yourself in a haze of wood smoke.

Outdoor pollution isn't the only problem. Indoor air pollution, in homes, offices, and factories, is a problem, too. Cigarettes aren't the only culprits. For example, we often don't consider paint fumes in a recently renovated area. We don't think about strong perfumes as we walk by the perfume sample counter at our local department store. Even the indoor ice rink has problems—the emissions from the Zamboni ice-resurfacing machine can cause respiratory symptoms.[2] Nitrogen dioxide levels within enclosed ice rinks may far exceed EPA air-quality standards.

Allergic triggers are also difficult to escape. Cat allergen, for example, is pervasive throughout our environment, even in places cats have never been. Cat allergen has been detected on brand-new beds (presumably from people lying down on them to try them out), and in the schools (as kids with cats at home bring the allergen in on their clothing).

Low-income communities often have the worst problems. Asthma problems are more common and more severe in low-income minority communities. Cockroaches can trigger asthma. Children who are allergic and live in roach-infested housing do the worst, according to the National Inner City Asthma Study.[3] Heating may be inadequate, making breathing problems worse in winter months. Or portable sources of heat may contribute to indoor air pollution. Burning anything inside the home can release pollutants—even "clean-burning" natural gas releases nitrogen oxides, which are well-known asthma triggers. A gas wall heater, a gas stove, or a kerosene heater will all adversely effect the quality of the indoor air.

Infestations with mice and rats can also lead to high levels of these allergens, which can trigger asthma. Crumbling wood, leaking walls and ceilings are another problem: the more moisture, the more mold growth. Polluting industries are often located in or near low-income communities.

Limiting pollution is not something that the industries will (or can) do voluntarily. After all, if one company invests heavily in pollution control, thereby driving up the price of its products, and another company pollutes to its heart's content, enabling it to sell its product much more cheaply, who is going to dominate the business? We can't just blame big business—even the most environmentally conscious of us will usually go straight for the cheaper product. Government regulation, then, is needed to impose uniform high standards to help keep the air in our communities clean.

I haven't even started to touch on handling the challenges of asthma if you are homeless—when it may be all you can do to find a place to sleep and food to eat. Keeping asthma in control may be much less of a priority when basic survival is such a challenge.

So, is it hopeless? Are these problems just too big?

Simple actions can yield big payoffs. Those asthma epidemics in Barcelona and New Orleans? No more. Now filters are used during loading to capture the soybean dust. These filters "cured" these asthma epidemics.[4] Simple action. Big payoff.

Yet when it comes to pollution, more and more of the blame is on us. Many of the early gains in air quality came from controlling what scientists call "point sources"—pollution coming from a single source, like a factory smokestack. Regulations have greatly reduced those emissions. Today the bigger problem is non-point source emissions—small sources that have a big cumulative impact. These are sources that are within the responsibility of ordinary citizens like you and me: our fireplaces, our barbecues, our cars.

Especially our cars. We could make a huge impact on air quality by driving smaller, more fuel-efficient and cleaner cars. Or better yet, using public transportation instead. Or a bicycle. Or even walk.

Controlling asthma, then, involves both personal and political actions. States that have passed laws limiting smoking in public buildings and workplaces have helped millions of people with asthma. Environmental controls on industry and automobiles have helped as well. I give credit to the American Lung Association for championing many lung health issues in our political process.

But we still have a long way to go. Remember, however, that as a parent of a child with asthma, you are not alone. In any group of 100 people, it is likely that you will find at least 5 to 15 who suffer from asthma. That's substantial. We can wield real power for change—if we're willing to put in the effort.

Sample Letter for School Personnel

To the teachers and staff at_____school:
_____has asthma.

His/her asthma symptoms include:
____Cough
____Wheeze
____Chest tightness
____Shortness of breath
____Rapid breathing
____Difficulty talking
____Decrease in peak flow rate
____Other:_____

His/her asthma can be brought on by:
____Smoke
____Dust
____Molds

_____Pollens
_____Animal dander (the shed skin of warm-blooded animals)
_____Viral infections (colds)
_____Exercise
_____Other:_____

Asthma Medicines:
She/he takes two types of medicines for asthma:

The first type is a *long-acting, controller* medication that s/he takes every day *to prevent* asthma from starting. This medication does not provide quick relief when an asthma flare-up starts.
My child's long-acting controller is:

_____

The second type is a *quick-relief* inhaler that s/he uses as needed for quick relief of asthma symptoms. This inhaler is can also be used right before exercise if needed to prevent exercise-induced asthma (if this is a problem).
My child's quick-relief inhaler is:

_____

Both of these medications are very safe if taken in recommended doses.

Green/Yellow/Red Zones:
I have attached a copy of the asthma management plan for my child, so that you can see what medications are needed when. I divide asthma control into green, yellow, and red zones (just like a traffic light).

Green zone means asthma is well controlled. Lung function is normal. *Green zone is where my child should be every day.*

Yellow zone is when asthma is just starting to kick up. Prompt action here can prevent a more severe attack. Allow my child to slow down. *Please let me know if my child is in the yellow zone.*

Red zone is danger zone. Please let me know as soon as possible when my child is in the red zone.
Be sure that my child gets his/her quick-relief inhaler right away.

There is an asthma emergency if:
    Difficulty breathing:
        Chest, abdomen, and/or neck pull in with breathing.
        Hunched over to breathe
        Very fast or rapid breathing
        Seems to struggle to breathe

Difficulty walking or talking due to asthma.
Lips or fingernails are turning gray or blue.
Peak Flow Rate below_____.

If you see any of these symptoms, get help IMMEDIATELY. **Call 911.** Then call me. While waiting for the ambulance, give my child his/her quick-relief inhaler.

Notes on use of the peak flow meter:
The peak flow meter can measure how tight or open the breathing tubes are. It can give a number that lets you know how bad (or good) my child's asthma is. The peak flow rate is affected by effort, how big the lungs are, and by how bad the asthma is. If done correctly, the peak flow rate can tell you if my child is in the green, yellow, or red zones.

For inhaled medications:
____My child knows the proper way to use asthma inhalers and shows appropriate judgment and responsibility about when to use them. She/he should be allowed to carry and use his/her asthma inhalers by himself/herself.
____Please supervise my child when s/he needs to use asthma medication.

Special instructions for my child:
_____
_____
_____
_____
_____
_____

Parent's Phone Numbers:
   Home: _____
   Work: _____
   Pager/Cell Phone: _____

Other Emergency Contact: _____
   Name: _____
   Relation: _____
   Phone Number: _____

_____
Parent's Signature   *Date*

_____
Physician's Signature   *Date*

HOW ASTHMA-FRIENDLY IS YOUR SCHOOL?

Children with asthma need proper support at school to keep their asthma under control and be fully active. Use the questions below to find out how well your school assists children with asthma:

Yes   No

1. Is your school *free of tobacco smoke* all of the time, including during school-sponsored events?

2. Does the school maintain *good indoor air quality?* Does it *reduce or eliminate allergens and irritants* that can make asthma worse? Allergens and irritants include pets with fur or feathers, mold, dust mites (for example, in carpets and upholstery), cockroaches, and strong odors or fumes from such products as pesticides, paint, perfumes, and cleaning chemicals.

3. Is there a *school nurse* in your school all day, every day? If not, is a nurse regularly available to the school to help write plans and give guidance for students with asthma about medicines, physical education, and field trips?

4. Can children take *medicines* at school as recommended by their doctor and parents? May children carry their own asthma medicines?

5. Does your school have an *emergency plan* for taking care of a child with a severe asthma episode (attack)? Is it made clear what to do? Who to call? When to call?

6. Does someone *teach school staff* about asthma, asthma management plans, and asthma medicines? Does someone *teach all students* about asthma and how to help a classmate who has it?

                                                      Yes   No

7. Do students have *good options for fully and*   _____ _____
   safely participating in physical education class
   and recess? (For example, do students have access
   to their medicine before exercise? Can they
   choose modified or alternative activities when
   medically necessary?)

If the answer to any question is no, students may be facing obstacles to asthma control. Asthma out of control can hinder a student's attendance, participation, and progress in school. School staff, health professionals, and parents can work together to remove obstacles and to promote students' health and education.

Asthma can be controlled; expect nothing less.

National Heart, Lung, and Blood Institute, National Asthma Education and Prevention Program, School Asthma Education Subcommittee

17

Complementary and Alternative Treatments

Studies on alternative and complementary treatments for asthma have been mixed.

Some of these approaches appear to help. Others fall into the "couldn't hurt" category. There's not much proof, at least not yet, that they're effective, but there's little chance that they'll cause harm—unless you use them as a *substitute* for proven medications. Still others are less effective than the drugs they supposedly replace, or have more side effects than conventional medications.

Some people will tell you that physicians are "opposed" to natural or alternative therapies. I'm neither for nor against them. I feel that they need to be judged the same way we judge any other treatment option: What does the evidence say? Are they safe? Effective? Do they have side effects? How do they stack up against other options? Will they interfere with other types of treatments?

A lot of times, the "evidence" for or against such treatments consists of testimonials and isolated case reports. I'm sure some people have seen dramatic improvements after using one or the other of these treatments. But the value of these kinds of reports—what scientific researchers call "anecdotal" evidence—is limited.

Here's why: You could pick out just about any "treatment"—say, peanut butter twice a day—and if you give it to enough people, some of those people will get better. Maybe it's because of the treatment. Or maybe it is for completely unrelated reasons—for example, because the seasons changed, or maybe the symptoms cleared up all on their own. Whatever the reason, these "successes" get a lot more attention than the failures (nobody gives testimonials about treatments that don't work). As a result, the treatments seem more successful than they really are.

It's kind of like what happens when you walk into the slot-machine room at a casino. All you hear are bells going off and money pouring out of the machines. It sounds as if everyone's winning. But if the casinos made buzzers go off every time someone *didn't* win, you'd draw a different conclusion.

So the only way to know for sure whether any treatment works—be it alternative or conventional—is to test it under scientific conditions. For example, we might set up two groups: one that gets the treatment and one that gets the conventional therapy. Then we compare results from the two groups. To reduce the chance that our results could be biased, we randomly assign subjects to treatment groups, otherwise the results might have more to do with how each person chose their treatment group than with the effect of the treatment. To further decrease the possibility of bias, we don't let the subjects or the investigators know which group a person is assigned to, otherwise our desire to prove something could influence the results.

Although things aren't always this simple in practice, these are the sorts of approaches we use to evaluate conventional treatments. It's also the kind of evidence the Food and Drug Administration insists on seeing before it will approve a new drug. As interest in alternative and complementary therapies grows, more and more of those therapies are being studied using this kind of approach.

But there's still a lot of work to be done in this area. By and large alternative medicine is where traditional (allopathic) medicine was in the 1800s. Back then, many treatments were based on a health care practitioner's experience, on what he was taught, or on the theory of disease that he happened to subscribe to. When we read some of those early case reports, they can be pretty hair-raising. Sometimes doctors came up with the right answers, but often as not they were just flat-out wrong.

For example, up until the nineteenth century, bleeding and purging were commonly prescribed treatments. Arsenic was used in remedies for problems as diverse as fever, heart disease, and indigestion. Tobacco was even recommended for asthma!

Little by little, researchers put these ideas to the test. They used the scientific methods that had been pioneered in disciplines like chemistry and physics.

It was slow going, for it turned out to be complicated to do such tests with living, breathing patients. Humans make lousy lab animals. They don't always do what they're told. They don't always tell the truth to researchers. They also come in an astonishing variety of ages, shapes, sizes, and conditions.

Looking back, the history of medical progress over the last century or so may seem like an orderly progression. But in reality, it involved a lot of false starts, wrong guesses, and head-scratching along the way.

So it may be a while until we build up the same track record with alternative treatments. Until then, we need to be cautious about drawing conclusions.

That said, there's a good chance that some of these treatments will ultimately improve asthma care. After all, most of the current conventional asthma treatments started as herbal remedies. For example:

- Strong coffee was commonly recommended for asthma in the eighteenth century. Theophylline (whose name means "tea leaves") is a close relative of caffeine and was first isolated from tea.
- A popular remedy first used in India, the leaves of *Datura stramonium* were often smoked for asthma. A related medicinal plant, *Atropa belladonna*, had been recognized by lay healers in America to have anti-asthma properties. The drug ipratropium (Atrovent) was designed to give the benefit of these herbal remedies without their often severe side effects.
- Khellin is another herbal remedy that had been used for centuries in the Middle East. It had lots of side effects, however; from it, the related anti-asthma compound cromolyn (Intal) was synthesized.
- The Chinese herb ma huang, which contains the active compound ephedrine, has been used for thousands of years as both a stimulant and for respiratory diseases. Albuterol (Ventolin, Proventil) acts by a similar mechanism, but with much fewer side effects.

So we know that many traditional herbal remedies do have active ingredients that work against asthma. But the simple fact that they're "natural" doesn't make them safer or gentler than drugs.

Oftentimes, in fact, the whole point of creating a synthetic drug is to gain the beneficial effect of a natural remedy while removing the harmful or unpleasant side effects. Each of the prescription medications mentioned above is much safer than their its related herbs. *Atropa belladonna* is also known as deadly nightshade, and it is a powerful poison. Ma huang can cause your blood pressure to go up and heart to race.

Fortunately, we're beginning to see more research being done examining complementary and alternative medicine treatments. In the near future we hope to have much better evidence to base our decisions on, and maybe some new asthma remedies will be recognized.

There have been some encouraging reports suggesting that some non-drug treatments may have a beneficial impact. Here's a summary of the available evidence:

The Best All-Natural Treatment

The best non-drug asthma remedy is to control asthma triggers in your environment. It's 100 percent natural, it has no side effects, and it's extremely effective. For example, I'd estimate that one-quarter of kids with asthma who live in homes with smokers could have their asthma *cured* if they lived in a smoke-free environment—and the remainder would have their asthma significantly improved. (See chapter 6 for more information on controlling asthma triggers in the home environment.)

Massage

Recently, a fascinating study compared massage with relaxation exercises for children with asthma. The children who got daily massages from their parents did significantly better than those who used relaxation exercise.[1]

This study raises some intriguing questions about the role of the parent-child relationship in asthma. Was the improvement a result of the massage itself? Did the massage promote greater physical relaxation? Or did the daily close physical contact between parent and child lead to a better relationship between them, so that the child became more cooperative and involved in her treatment?

We still don't know the answer to that one. But if a massage a day works, I'm all for it. I can't see a downside. And who knows—maybe after parents come home from a hard day's work, the kids will return the favor.

Meditation

Meditation is useful in coping with chronic illness. It reduces stress and improves one's sense of personal well-being. Though I haven't seen any studies of meditation directly related to asthma, I wouldn't be surprised to find that this technique has a positive effect. A key component of some meditation techniques involves focusing on your breathing. That can help us to gain a better awareness of what's going on in our bodies. It may help us get better at identifying early signs of trouble and to know when we need to use a short-acting inhaler.

We've seen some patients take a meditative approach to using their inhalers. Instead of viewing the inhaler as an unwelcome intrusion, they use it as an opportunity to take a step back and get in touch with what their bodies and lungs are telling them. In fact, the proper breathing technique for using an inhaler (see chapter 12) is similar to the type of breathing that's practiced in some forms of meditation.

Vitamins

Vitamin C may have some beneficial effect on asthma, but the evidence is sketchy. Some studies have found that low dietary vitamin C intake is associated with an increased risk of asthma. Other studies, however, found no association.

I'd put vitamin C in the "couldn't hurt" category—as long as you don't go overboard. Probably the best vitamin C supplement is in the natural form of fresh fruits. If you give your child a pill-form vitamin C supplement, I would suggest that you avoid megadoses. The recommended daily allowance is fine; megadoses may increase the body's metabolism of vitamin C, which could cause problems if the supplement is stopped suddenly.

Fish Oil

There is also some suggestion that a diet high in fish oil may help asthma. At this point, however, the evidence is preliminary, and I think the jury's still out on this one. However, if you like oily fish, this sort of evidence lets you feel good about having it in your diet. That's more than I could say about hamburgers and french fries.

Chiropractic

Thorough studies have shown no benefit for the use of chiropractic in the treatment of asthma.[2]

. . .

The bottom line: massage, vitamin C, and fish oil may be of some benefit. Herbs potent enough to affect asthma carry significant side effects. Chiropractic does not appear to be of any help in asthma.

None of these approaches can fully substitute for asthma medications. Use them alongside proven asthma medications, not instead of them. And remember that "natural" compounds can have risks and side effects as well. Be sure to discuss with your doctor any complementary/ alternative remedies that you are using or considering.

18

The Future of Asthma Care

Is the revolution over for those of us who study and treat asthma?

Hardly. I've seen our entire approach to asthma treatment change over the last fifteen years. Yet I still think of my dean's admonition that half of what we know will turn out be wrong. Fifteen years from now, we could see yet another revolution in the field.

Most of the advances we've seen so far have addressed how we *treat* asthma. But we're still scratching the surface. The next big areas will be how to *prevent* asthma and how to *cure* it. Though there are many theories, we really do not know what causes some people (and not others) to have asthma. Do infections make things better or worse? There is good evidence pointing in both directions. Is allergen exposure at an early age good or bad? What is it about our Western lifestyle that causes asthma?

I expect that we'll see continued refinements in our approach to treatment, with newer, better drugs, with even fewer side effects and more convenience. For example, though we have very good, very safe medication to control mild to moderate asthma, severe asthma remains a challenge. We're still asking patients to manage complex drug regimens. We could make drugs more efficient. Even the best of the preparations are able to get only a small part of the dose into the lungs.

What's Coming in Drugs

In my view, the ideal asthma medication would:

* Effectively block the underlying inflammation that causes asthma
* Work quickly
* Be easy to use
* Still be effective even if used only occasionally
* Have no or minimal short-term side effects
* Have no long-term side effects
* Be safe for children
* Not cost much

Researchers are looking for new medications with these and other benefits. The stakes are huge: People spend a lot of money every year buying asthma medications, so a new breakthrough could be worth billions to the company that develops it.

Unfortunately, that also means that drug companies have a vested interest in promoting "breakthrough" drugs that, well, really may not represent all that much of a breakthrough.

Let me share some words of wisdom that my teachers shared with me about new drugs: Be neither the first nor the last to jump on board. Before release, a new drug is studied in hundreds, possibly thousands of people. After release, it may be used by millions of people. Uncommon, but potentially severe, side effects may only be seen once a new medicine is in wide release.

The absence of evidence is not the same as evidence of absence. Many a new drug has come on the market with the hype that it is very safe, only for problems to crop up later. Seldane (terfenadine), for example, was a very popular non-sedating antihistamine when it first came out. Only after millions of people had taken the drug did we find that it could cause irregular heart rhythm and death.[1] It may only be possible to find some problems after large numbers of people have used the drug.

You have to balance risk and benefit. If your child has very severe asthma and treatment is causing lots of side effects, it may be more worth your while to be among the first to try a promising new medicine. On the other hand, if your child has mild to moderate asthma that is well controlled with minimal side effects of treatment, you can easily afford to watch and wait to see what happens.

So with those caveats in mind, let's take a look at what's in development. Researchers are focusing on three key strategies:

* Improving delivery systems (such as inhalers) to make old drugs work better with fewer side effects
* Creating new drugs that have the beneficial action of the old drugs but with more potency and fewer side effects
* Finding entirely new classes of drugs that have anti-asthma properties

Asthma Drug Delivery Systems

One key area of research focuses on creating metered-dose inhalers that don't use CFCs (which are bad for the ozone layer) and, equally important, get more of the medication dispersed into very small particles that can get into the lungs. As you recall from chapter 5, today's metered-dose inhalers create a mixture of particle sizes, and the big particles don't get past the mouth and throat. Medicine should be more effective at lower doses if more gets to the lungs. A lower, but more effective, dose would pose less risk of side effects.

A related effort is to create a sort of cross between a metered-dose inhaler and a nebulizer, which can take liquid medicine and make it into a single puff of mist without having to use any kind of chemical propellant.

A third area of research is looking at how to create devices that can take a dose of dry powder medicine and make it into a fine mist, one that can stay suspended in the air long enough so that even a small infant could breathe it in. The new device would be sort of a cross between a dry powder inhaler and a nebulizer—and this would be easier to use.

Asthma Drugs

New Corticosteroids

Several pharmaceutical companies are looking at creating new inhaled corticosteroid medications. The goal is to design one with a high level of action at the breathing tubes, but either minimal absorption from the breathing tubes into the body and/or minimal action elsewhere in the body. Here, again, the goal is to reduce side effects, which could potentially allow us to use higher doses in more severe cases.

Antibodies to IgE

Immunoglobulin E (IgE) is an antibody that is associated with allergy and asthma. People with severe allergies and asthma often have high levels of IgE. Maybe if we could remove some of the IgE, we could have an anti-asthma effect. A genetically engineered mouse has been created that can make antibodies against human IgE. The mouse was further tinkered with so that these antibodies look like human antibodies—not mouse antibodies.

Preliminary studies suggest that use of this "humanized" mouse anti-IgE can reduce the level of this asthma-causing IgE antibody, and that doing this does have a modest anti-asthma effect.[2] More work is needed on how to deliver the medicine, and long-term safety needs investigation.

Theophylline

As we've seen, this drug has a modest anti-asthma action, but its caffeinelike side effects sometimes make it unpleasant to use, and overdoses can cause severe problems. Researchers are investigating whether it is possible to construct a drug that expands on the benefit of theophylline but reduces the side effects.

Toward Prevention and Cure

What causes a person to have asthma?

The factors that cause asthma may be very different from the factors that trigger asthma once it's already present. For example, some types of air pollution make people who have asthma cough and wheeze. But that doesn't mean that this same pollution can *give* asthma to someone who doesn't have it.

Finding the ultimate causes of asthma isn't easy. After all, you can't give people things that might cause them to develop asthma, then wait to see if they get asthma or not. So we need to look at natural exposures for clues to causation. We can look at natural experiments, for example the different lifestyles of people in East and West Germany before and after reunification (and being surprised to find asthma and allergy less common in the more polluted East Germany).[3] We can compare people in different parts of the world—and notice that asthma is much more common in westernized societies. What is it about our Western lifestyle that brings out allergies and asthma?

A powerful research method is to follow people in detail, from birth through early adulthood, getting as much information about them as possible as they grow up, and then looking back to see what was different about the individuals who developed asthma and the ones who did not. Studies, such as the Tucson Children's Respiratory Study, which was started about fifteen years ago, are starting to yield some exciting results. Contrary to what we expected to find, new research suggests:

- If you start life with low lung function, you may have a wheezing illness a time or two as an infant, but it is possible that you will not go on to have asthma as an older child.[4]
- If you are in day care as an infant, you will probably get more colds as an infant, but your risk of asthma later in life may actually be decreased.[5] If you have asthma already, however, nothing will set off an attack like a viral infection.
- If you grow up with pets at home, your risk of developing asthma may be decreased. However, if you have asthma already and are allergic to the pet, your asthma will almost certainly be worse.[6]
- If you grow up on a farm, your risk of developing allergies may be decreased.[7]

Nobody's quite sure what all this means. But one intriguing possibility is that people who are exposed to these kinds of triggers very early in life may be less likely to develop asthma. In other words, the same things that cause asthma attacks in people who already have the disease may prevent the disease in others.

The theory is that infancy is a critical time for the development of the immune system. An infant's immune system can develop in one of two ways. It can develop brisk responses to bacteria and viruses in the environment. But if the infections are not around, the immune system may develop in another way—causing allergies and asthma.[8] Keep in mind that this is just a theory, evidence is just starting to come in. Also, of course, control of severe infections has dramatically reduced infant mortality. And there is *no* evidence to suggest that any of the routine childhood immunizations have any effect (one way or the other) on asthma or allergy.

A word of caution, however, in this rapidly changing world: Many more provocative theories and strongly held opinions exist than strong evidence to support them.

19

Frequently Asked Questions

Will my child grow out of asthma?

The short answer is maybe.

Lots of infants will have a wheezing episode with a viral respiratory infection. Some will have only one or two, thereby growing out of it; some will go on to have many episodes of chest tightness. If there is a family history of allergies and asthma, there is a better chance that the wheezing and chest tightness will persist.

Adolescence is also a time of change. For many children asthma gets better. For others, it gets worse. The more severe the asthma was before adolescence, the less likely the child will "grow out of it."

But even when asthma improves during the teenage years, it may be more of an intermission than a final act. Your best lung function is at about age sixteen. After that, it starts to decline. Sometimes asthma that is "outgrown" in adolescence returns later in life. Generally, the milder the asthma is, the greater the chance that an adolescent will "grow out of it."

Some people believe that waiting to outgrow the asthma is how to manage it. I do not share that belief. You need to deal with what you have now to obtain your best lung function—now. Keeping your asthma in good control now can make it easier to control later.[1] Years of poorly controlled asthma may cause permanent changes to the breathing tubes.

Do I need to restrict my child's activities?

Though restricting activities may be one way to cope with poorly controlled asthma, it is a poor way to cope with life. *A full, active life is important for a healthy mind and body.* Regular exercise is important for the health of the heart and the lungs. Participation in sports is important for the social development of the child. If a person is meant to be a superstar athlete, asthma shouldn't hold him or her back.

Exercise-induced asthma can be managed (see pages 51–52). The first principle is to keep the underlying asthma in as good control as possible—by controlling asthma triggers and, if needed, by using an inhaled anti-inflammatory (preventive) medicine every day. Adherence to this first principle alone will often dramatically improve exercise tolerance. The second principle is to use a quick reliever (like albuterol) shortly before going out to exercise, compete, or vigorously play.

If asthma is starting to act up (peak flows in yellow zone), have your child take it easy. The lungs are not in the best shape to handle vigorous activity. On yellow zone days, consider sending a note to your child's teacher suggesting that your child be allowed to refrain from vigorous activity.

What athletic activities are best for children with asthma?

Ten years ago I would have emphatically replied, "Swimming," because it's the athletic activity least likely to trigger asthma. However, with good strategies now available to control asthma, the choice of sports activities need not be limited. The advice that I give for parents of children with asthma is the same as for children without asthma: Choose activities that your child enjoys and are reasonably safe.

Are inhaled steroids harmful?

Inhaled corticosteroids in low to moderate doses have an excellent safety record. My colleagues and I have treated thousands of patients with these drugs. Out of these thousands of patients, very few have had problems with hoarseness of the voice. A couple of patients who did not use a spacer or rinse their mouth got oral thrush (white plaques on the cheeks due to yeast). One patient of mine had problems with the inhaler causing cough (due to the "inactive" ingredients in the inhaler). And there have been a handful of patients on moderate doses of inhaled steroids who had slight slowing of their growth rate. Instead of their height being a little bit above average, it was a little bit below average, perhaps half an inch or so. Very high doses of inhaled corticosteroids (800 micrograms per day or more) can cause side effects that are more significant (see chapter 7).

Keep in mind that poorly controlled asthma has plenty of side effects: trouble with exercise, school, and work; sedentary lifestyles; difficulty sleeping. To say nothing of permanent changes to the breathing tubes from years of chronic inflammation.

My baby cries whenever I try to give him inhaled medicine.
What should I do?

Though none of us like to hear a baby cry, it's not a bad thing when it comes to getting inhaled medicines into the lung. When a baby cries, a deep breath is taken, which helps the medicine go in. Inhaled medicine can be given to a crying infant, as well as a quiet baby.

It seems that I always have to fight with my child about taking
asthma medicine. What can I do?

This is one of the big challenges in raising a child—how do you get them to do what they are supposed to do? Everyone has their own strategies that work for them; however, let me share with you a few strategies that have worked for the parents of my patients.

- Praise. Be sure to notice when your child takes the medicine well. Nothing works to encourage good behavior like some well-timed praise.
- Prioritize. Pick just two or three behaviors that you want to change.
- Use positive reinforcement. If the medicine is taken well, give your child a gold star. Make the gold stars negotiable: three stars equal a small gift or privilege, twenty stars equal a more valuable gift or privilege.

- Teach your child about what the medicine does, how it works, and why he needs to take it.
- Make it part of the daily routine. Link it to brushing teeth, getting dressed, or eating meals.
- Keep a calendar. Write when the medicine is taken on the calendar. You can record peak flow rates also.
- Give your child choices. Does she want to use the blue spacer or the yellow spacer? What story does he want you to read to him after he takes his inhaler (or while he takes his nebulizer treatment)?
- Ask your doctor how you can simplify your child's asthma care regimen.
- If the child complains about the taste of the inhaler, ask your doctor about other medicines that don't taste as bad.

My child insists on taking his medicine by himself.
How can I know if he is really doing it?

Here are two ways to tell: One, he gets good outcomes. That means asthma stays well controlled. School attendance and sports participation is not limited by asthma. There is no cough, no wheeze, and peak flow rates are staying in the top of the green zone.

Two, the preventive medicine gets used up in a timely fashion (see chart on page 80) and quick-acting symptom relief medicine is needed infrequently. If your child is doing well and the asthma is well controlled, quick-acting symptom relievers like albuterol should be needed infrequently (a puff or two before exercise really should be about it). If asthma is well controlled, a canister of albuterol (or other quick-acting symptom reliever) should last three to four months at least. If you need to get refills more often, you need to investigate what is going on.

I have heard about asthma camps. What are they?
How do I get my child into one?

Asthma camps are summer camps for children with asthma. Many American Lung Association chapters run asthma camps. They give kids a chance to meet and make friends with other children who have asthma. They also teach kids about their lungs and asthma. And they give kids a chance to just have some fun in a safe environment.

For more information about asthma camps call your local lung association chapter at 800-LUNG-USA.

Does stress cause asthma?

No. If stress caused asthma, asthma would be a lot more common than it is. Probably the least useful thing to hear is, "If only you would learn to relax, then you wouldn't have asthma."

However, stress can make asthma that is already present worse. Relaxation exercises help a person who has asthma.

It seems that my child goes quickly from almost normal to a severe asthma flare-up. What can I do to prevent this?

Usually this pattern tells us that the child is living right on the edge of control. It's like living on a cliff. One false step and down you go.

To avoid falling off the cliff, move away!

First, discuss with your child's doctor the use of a daily preventive medication to make the breathing tubes less sensitive (see chapter 7, "Managing the Breathing Tubes").

Second, figure out your child's early-warning signs, and take prompt, aggressive action when they appear. Your child's early-warning signs may be different from others', so think about what happened 12 to 24 hours before your child's last flare-up. Did she get a cold? An ear infection? Did peak flow rates start to go down? Was your child exposed to smoke? A cat? Did it start with a cough? A tickle in the throat? Did he have trouble sleeping at night?

Despite everything that I have done to control the asthma, there is still frequent coughing, wheezing, and chest tightness. What can I do?

The most common reasons for poorly controlled asthma are (in no particular order):

- Living with an asthma trigger
- Not using (or not using enough) anti-inflammatory medication to prevent asthma
- Poor technique in using inhaled medications (very little of it is getting to the lungs)
- Complicating medical conditions that can trigger asthma (such as sinus infections and acid reflux from the stomach)
- Mimickers: symptoms caused by something other than asthma

If you have addressed all of these issues and asthma is still not controlled, *this may be the time to see an asthma specialist—a pediatric pulmonologist or allergist.*

My child hates to use asthma inhalers at school; it makes him feel "different." How can I deal with this?

If asthma is well controlled, your child shouldn't need to use inhalers routinely at school. Control asthma triggers, monitor peak flow rates, and use inhaled preventive medication daily to keep asthma in good control.

If exercise-induced asthma at school is a problem (and asthma is otherwise in good control), there are two strategies. The best is to use one to two puffs of a quick-relief medicine like albuterol (Ventolin, Proventil) just before exercise. The other option is to use a long-acting symptom reliever like salmeterol (Serevent) in the morning before school. The first option is better.

If your child does need to use an inhaler at school, he can use it in the office, locker room, or the bathroom so he's not in front of the other kids. A better strategy, I think, is to help him become comfortable with using it anywhere, anytime. Often if he explains to the other kids about his asthma and why he needs the medicine, classmates will be supportive and understanding. They may want to do a book report or a science project on asthma.

Are short-haired pets less allergenic?

It's not the hair that's the allergen; it's the shed skin (also called dander). Short-haired pets and pets that don't shed can cause just as much of an allergy problem as their long-haired brethren.

Why does asthma seem so much worse at night?

Asthma *is* worse at night. I have had parents tell me of being up struggling with their child's asthma all night, but when they brought the child into the doctor early that afternoon, they felt embarrassed and patronized when the doctor said that their child looked fine. The experienced parent knows that the child may make it through the day okay, but will often face another struggle the following night.

The reason, as much as we understand it, is circadian rhythms. Lung function is normally lowest at night, highest at midday. So the lungs are most vulnerable to asthma in the middle of the night.

Exposure to certain asthma triggers may also be the greatest at night. The bed is a haven for dust mites. See pages 42–43 for information on how to control exposure to dust mites.

How do I communicate with my doctor about my child's asthma?

It's important to use terms that your doctor understands. Measure your child's peak flow rate when she is having trouble (and see how far down it is from her personal best). Describe any difficulty in breathing that your child had. Measure the breathing rate (number of breaths in one minute). And describe any breathing noises your child was making.

Taking all those puffs is hard. What can be done?

With the current generation of asthma medications, it is unusual for anyone to need more than four puffs at a time. Often with high-potency medications you can work with your doctor to get the number of puffs even lower. It's important that you tell your doctor that reducing the number of puffs your child takes is important for you. Doctors tend to assume that if you don't raise the issue, everything's fine.

The other strategy is to make taking the asthma inhalers a pleasant, relaxing experience. Suggest that your child pay attention to the breath. Take a slow deep breath. Imagine how the air combined with the medicine is helping the lungs and body feel better. Imagine the inflammation of the breathing tubes just melting away. Or imagine that you are on a beautiful beach, taking in the clean ocean air. Feel the stress, and the asthma, leave your body as you breathe out. Notice how much better it makes you feel.

What should I bring to a visit with my child's doctor?

- Bring a copy of your child's asthma diary, so the doctor can get an accurate picture of how your child has been doing.
- Bring all medicines, so your doctor knows exactly what your child has been taking.
- Bring your child's spacer devices and peak flow meter. Technique is important for the effective use of these devices. It is important that your child's health care provider check how these devices are used.
- It is important to have the people who make decisions about the child's care (Mom, Dad, Grandmother, etc.) at the visit so they hear the same thing, are all on the same page, and all work off the same plan.

Notes

ABBREVIATIONS

Allergy Asthma Proc — *Allergy and Asthma Proceedings*
Am J Epidemiol — *American Journal of Epidemiology*
Am J Respir Crit Care Med — *American Journal of Respiratory and Critical Care Medicine*
Am Rev Respir Dis — *American Review of Respiratory Diseases*
Ann Allergy Asthma Immunol — *Annals of Allergy, Asthma, and Immunology*
Arch Environ Health — *Archives of Environmental Health*
Arch Intern Med — *Archives of Internal Medicine*
BMJ — *British Medical Journal*
Clin Exp Allergy — *Clinical and Experimental Allergy*
Clin Ther — *Clinical Therapeutics*
Eur Respir J — *European Respiratory Journal*
J Allergy Clin Immunol — *Journal of Allergy and Clinical Immunology*
J Asthma — *Journal of Asthma*
J Pediatr — *Journal of Pediatrics*
N Engl J Med — *New England Journal of Medicine*
NIH — *National Institutes of Health*
Pediatr Pulmonol — *Pediatric Pulmonology*
Pediatr Res — *Pediatric Research*
Respir Med — *Respiratory Medicine*

Introduction: The Mystery Epidemic

1. National Heart, Lung, and Blood Institute. *Data Fact Sheet: Asthma Statistics.* January 1999.

2. von Mutius, E. Martinez, F. D., Fritzsch, C., Nicolai, T., Roell, G., Thiemann, H. H. Prevalence of asthma and atopy in two areas of West and East Germany. *Am J Respir Crit Care Med* 149 (1994): 358–64.

3. Ball, T. M., Castro-Rodriguez, J. A., Griffith, K. A., Holberg, C. J., Martinez, E. D., Wright, A. L. Siblings, day-care attendance, and the risk of asthma and wheezing during childhood. *N Engl J Med* 343 (2000): 538–43.

4. Remes, S. T., Castro-Rodriguez, J. A., Holberg, C. J., Martinez, F. D., Taussig, L., Wright, A. Pet exposure in infancy and wheeze and asthma in childhood (abstract). *Am J Respir Crit Care Med* 161 (March 2000): A704.

2: Taking Control

1. Ko, T. Kaiser Permanente Northern California Region Department of Quality and Utilization. Personal communication, 1999. Data are from Kaiser Permanente Northern California Region hospitals, children 0–17 years. Data are adjusted for service population.

3: Welcome to the Revolution

1. Larsen, G. L. Asthma in children. *N Engl J Med* 326 (1992): 1540–45.

2. Laitinen, L. A., Heino, M., Laitinen, A., Kava, T., Haahtela, T. Damage of the airway epithelium and bronchial reactivity in patients with asthma. *Am Rev Respir Dis* 131 (1985): 599–606; Beasley, R., Roche, W. R., Roberts, J. A., Holgate, S. T. Cellular events in the bronchi in mild asthma and after bronchial provocation. *Am Rev Respir Dis* 139 (1989): 806–17.

3. Littenberg, B., Gluck, E. H. A controlled trial of methylprednisolone in the emergency treatment of acute asthma. *N Engl J Med* 314 (1986): 150–52; Tal, A., Levy, N., Bearman, J. E. Methylprednisolone therapy for acute asthma in infants and toddlers: a controlled clinical trial. *Pediatrics* 86 (1990): 350–56.

4. Haahtela, T., Jarvinen, M., Kava, T., Kiviranta, K., Koskinen, S., Lehtonen, K., Nikander, K., Persson, T., Reinikainen, K., Selroos, O., et al. Comparison of a beta 2-agonist, terbutaline, with an inhaled corticosteroid, budesonide, in newly detected asthma. *N Engl J Med* 325 (1991): 388–92; van Essen-Zandvliet, E. E., Hughes, M. D., Waalkens, H. J., Duiverman, E. J., Pocock, S. J., Kerrebijn, K. F. Effects of 22 months of treatment with inhaled corticosteroids and/or beta-2-agonists on lung function, airway responsiveness, and symptoms in children with asthma. *Am Rev Respir Dis* 146 (1992): 547–54.

5. NIH. *National Asthma Education and Prevention Program Expert Panel Report: Guidelines for the Diagnosis and Management of Asthma.* Publication no. 91–3642. Revised 1997 as *Expert Panel Report 2: Guidelines for*

the Diagnosis and Management of Asthma. Publication No. 97–4051 (April 1997). Available for free download on the Internet at http://www.nhlbi.nih. gov/guidelines/asthma/asthgdln.htm.

6. Sears, M. R., Taylor, D. R., Print, C. G., Lake, D. C., Li, Q. Q., Flannery, E. M., Yates, D. M., Lucas, M. K., Herbison, G. P. Regular inhaled beta-agonist treatment in bronchial asthma. *Lancet* 336 (1990): 1391–96.

7. Lieu, T. A., Quesenberry, C. P., Sorel, M. E., Mendoza, G. R., Leong, A. B. Computer-based models to identify high-risk children with asthma. *Am J Respir Crit Care Med* 157 (1998): 1173–80.

8. Spitzer, W. O., Suissa, S., Ernst, P., Horwitz, R. I., Habbick, B., Cockcroft, D., Boivin, J. F., McNutt, M., Buist, A. S., Rebuck, A. S. The use of beta-agonists and the risk of death and near death from asthma. *N Engl J Med* 326 (1992): 501–6.

9. Busse, W. W., Chervinsky, P., Condemi, J., Lumry, W. R., Petty, T. L., Rennard, S., Townley, R. G. Budesonide delivered by Turbuhaler is effective in a dose-dependent fashion when used in the treatment of adult patients with chronic asthma. *J Allergy Clin Immunol* 101 (1998): 457–63.

10. Greening, A. P., Ind, P. W., Northfield, M., Shaw, G. Added salmeterol versus higher-dose corticosteroid in asthma patients with symptoms on existing inhaled corticosteroid. *Lancet* 344 (1994): 219–24.

11. Bousquet, J., Jeffery, P. K., Busse, W. W., Johnson, M., Vignola, A. M. Asthma: From bronchoconstriction to airways inflammation and remodeling. *Am Rev Respir Crit Care Med* 161 (2000): 1720–45.

12. Agertoft, L., Pedersen, S. Effects of long-term treatment with an inhaled corticosteroid on growth and pulmonary function in asthmatic children. *Respir Med* 88 (1994): 373–81.

13. Selroos, O., Pietinalho, A., Löfroos, A., Riska, H. Effect of early vs late intervention with inhaled corticosteroids in asthma. *Chest* 108 (1995): 1228–34.

4. An Ounce of Prevention

1. Smillie, J. G. *Can Physicians Manage the Quality and Costs of Health Care: The Story of the Permanente Medical Group*. New York: McGraw-Hill, 1991.

2. National Heart, Lung, and Blood Institute. Data Fact Sheet: Asthma Statistics. January 1999.

3. Lieu, T. A., Quesenberry, C. P., Sorel, M. E., Mendoza, G. R., Leong, A. B. Computer-based models to identify high-risk children with asthma. *Am J Respir Crit Care Med* 157 (1998): 1173–80.

6. Managing the Environment

1. Capra, A., Jensvold, N., Chi, F., Lieu, T., Farber, H., Lozano, P., Finkelstein, J., et al. *Asthma Care Quality Assessment Study*. Unpublished data.

2. Farber, H. J., Wattigney, W., Berenson, G. Trends in asthma prevalence: The Bogalusa heart study. *Ann Allergy Asthma Immunol* 78 (1997): 265–69.

3. Questions adapted from U.S. Public Health Service, "You Can Quit Smoking," Consumer Guide. June 2000. http://www.surgeongeneral.gov/tobacco/consquits.htm.

4. Adapted from "Help for Smokers: Ideas to Help You Quit," based on the U.S. Public Health Service, Tobacco Cessation Guideline. Rockville, Md.: Agency for Healthcare Research and Quality. June 2000. http://www.ahrq.gov/consumer/helpsmok.htm.

5. Rosenstreich, D. L., Eggleston, P., Kattan, M., Baker, D., Slavin, R. G., Gergen, P., et al. The role of cockroach allergy and exposure to cockroach allergen in causing morbidity among inner-city children with asthma. *N Eng J Med* 336 (1997): 1356–63.

6. Gergen, P. J., Mortimer, K. M., Eggleston, P. A., Rosenstreich, D., Mitchell, H., Ownby, D., et al. Results of the national cooperative inner-city asthma study (NCICAS) environmental intervention to reduce cockroach allergen exposure in inner-city homes. *J Allergy Clin Immunol* 103 (1999): 501–6.

7. Solomon, W. R., Platts-Mills, T. A. E. "Aerobiology and Inhalant Allergens," in E. Middleton, ed., *Allergy: Principles and Practice*, 5th ed. St. Louis, Mo.: Mosby-Year Book, 1998.

8. Infante-Rivard, C. Childhood asthma and indoor environmental risk factors. *Am J Epidemiol* 137 (1993): 834–44; Dekker, C., Dales, R., Bartlett, S., Brunekreef, B., Zwanenburg, H. Childhood asthma and the indoor environment. *Chest* 100 (1991): 922–26.

9. Burks, A. W., Mallory, S. B., Williams, L. W. et al. Atopic dermatitis: Clinical relevance of food hypersensitivity reactions. *J Pediatr* 113 (1988): 447–51.

10. Weiler, J. M., Layton, T., Hunt, M. Asthma in United States Olympic athletes who participated in the 1996 Summer Games. *J Allergy Clin Immunol* 102 (1998): 722–26.

11. Weiler, J. M., Ryan, E. J. Asthma in United States Olympic athletes who participated in the 1998 Olympic Winter Games. *J Allergy Clin Immunol* 106 (2000): 267–71.

7. *Managing the Breathing Tubes*

1. Farber, H. J., Lieu, T. A., Lozano, P., Capra, A. M., Chi, F., Jensvold, N. G., Finkelstein, J. A. Parent misunderstanding of role of asthma medication in a Medicaid managed care population (abstract). *Pediatr Res* 47 (2000): 477A.

2. Barnes, P. J., Pedersen, S., Busse, W. W. Efficacy and safety of inhaled corticosteroids: New developments. *Am J Respir Crit Care Med* 157 (1998): S1–S53.

3. Agertoft, L., Pedersen, S. Bone mineral density in children with asthma receiving long-term treatment with inhaled budesonide. *Am J Respir Crit Care Med* 157 (1998): 178–83.

4. Cumming, R. G., Mitchell, P., Leeder S. R. Use of inhaled corticosteroids and the risk of cataracts. *N Engl J Med* 337 (1997): 8–14.

5. Simons, F. E., Persuad, M. P., Gillespie, C. A., Cheang, M., Shuckett, E. P. Absence of posterior subcapsular cataracts in young patients treated with inhaled glucocorticoids. *Lancet* 342 (1993): 776–78; Agertoft, L., Larsen, F. E., Pedersen, S. Posterior subcapsular cataracts, bruises, and hoarseness in children with asthma receiving long-term treatment with inhaled budesonide. *Eur Respir J* 12 (1998):130–35; Abuekteish, F., Kirkpatrick, J. N., Russell, G. Posterior subcapsular cataract and inhaled corticosteroid therapy. *Thorax* 50 (1995): 674–66.

6. Pedersen, S., O'Byrne, P. A comparison of the efficacy and safety of inhaled corticosteroids in asthma. *Allergy* 52 (Suppl 39) (1997): 1–34; Wolthers, O. D., Pedersen, S. Growth of asthmatic children during treatment with budesonide: A double-blind trial. *BMJ* 303 (1991): 163–65.

7. Simons, E. E. R., et al. A Comparison of beclomethasone, salmeterol, and placebo in children with asthma. *N Engl J Med* 337 (1997): 1659–65.

8. Childhood Asthma Management Program Research Group. Long-term effects of budesonide or nedocromil in children with asthma. *N Engl J Med* 343 (2000): 1054–63.

9. Agertoft, L., Pedersen, S. Effect of long term treatment with inhaled budesonide on adult height in children with asthma. *N Engl J Med* 343 (2000): 1064–69.

10. Busse, W. W., Chervinsky, P., Condemi, J., Lumry, W. R., Petty, T. L., Rennard, S., Townley, R. G. Budesonide delivered by Turbuhaler is effective in a dose-dependent fashion when used in the treatment of adult patients with chronic asthma. *J Allergy Clin Immunol* 101 (1998): 457–63.

11. "Periodic Assessment and Monitoring: Essential for Asthma Management," in *National Asthma Education and Prevention Program Expert Panel Report 2: Guidelines for the Diagnosis and Management of Asthma*. Publication no. 97–4051 (April 1997).

12. Agertoft, L., Pedersen, S. Effects of long-term treatment with an inhaled corticosteroid on growth and pulmonary function in asthmatic children. *Respir Med* 88 (1994): 373–81.

13. Suissa, S., Ernst, P., Benayoun, S., Baltzan, M., Cai, B. Low-dose inhaled corticosteroids and the prevention of death from asthma. *N Engl J Med* 343 (2000): 332–36.

14. NIH. "Estimated Comparative Daily Dosages for Inhaled Corticosteroids," *National Asthma Education and Prevention Program Expert Panel Report 2: Guidelines for the Diagnosis and Management of Asthma*. Publication no. 97–4051 (April 1997).

15. O'Donohue, W. J., et al. Guidelines for the use of nebulizers in the home and at domiciliary sites: Report of a consensus conference. *Chest* 109 (1996): 814–20.

16. Greening, A. P., Ind, P. W., Northfield, M., Shaw, G. Added salmeterol versus higher-dose corticosteroid in asthma patients with symptoms on existing inhaled corticosteroid. *Lancet* 344 (1994): 219–24; Evans, D. J., Taylor, D. A., Zetterstrom, O., Chung, K. F., O'Connor, B. J., Barnes, P. J. A comparison of low-dose inhaled budesonide plus theophylline and high-dose inhaled budesonide for moderate asthma. *N Engl J Med* 337 (1997): 1412–48.

17. Greening, A. P., et al. See note 16.

18. Ramage, L., Lipworth, B. J., Ingram, O. G., Cree, I. A., Dhillon, D. P. Reduced protection against exercise induced bronchoconstriction after chronic dosing with salmeterol. *Respir Med* 88 (1994): 363–38; Cheung, D., Timmers, M. C., Zwinderman, A. H., Bel, E. H., Dijkman, J. H., Sterk, P. J. Long-term effects of a long-acting beta 2-adrenoceptor agonist, salmeterol, on airway hyperresponsiveness in patients with mild asthma. *N Engl J Med* 327 (1992): 1198–203; Cockcroft, D. W., McParland, C. P., Britto, S. A., Swystun, V. A., Rutherford, E. C. Regular inhaled salbutamol and airway responsiveness to allergen. *Lancet* 342 (1993): 833–37.

19. Evans, D. J., Taylor, D. A., Zetterstrom, O., Chung, K. F., O'Connor, B. J., Barnes, P. J. A comparison of low-dose inhaled budesonide plus theophylline and high-dose inhaled budesonide for moderate asthma. *N Engl J Med* 337 (1997): 1412–18.

20. Abramson, M. J., Puy, R. M., Weiner, J. M. Is allergen immunotherapy effective in asthma?: A meta-analysis of randomized controlled trials. *Am J Respir Crit Care Med* 151 (1995): 969–74.

21. Platts-Mills, T. A. E. "Immunotherapy in the Treatment of Asthma," in B. D. Rose, ed., *Up to Date Version 8.1.* Wellesley, Mass.: Up to Date, Inc., 2000.

22. American Academy of Pediatrics Committee on Drugs. Use of codeine- and dextromethorphan-containing cough remedies in children. *Pediatrics* 99 (1997): 918–20.

8. Managing Flare-Ups

1. Kikuchi, Y., Okabe, S., Tamura, G., Hida, W., Homma, M., Shirato, K., Takishima, T. Chemosensitivity and perception of dyspnea in patients with a history of near-fatal asthma. *N Engl J Med* 330 (1994): 1329–34.

2. Chapman, K. R., Verbeek, P. R, White, J. G., Rebuck, A. S. Effect of a short course of prednisone in the prevention of early relapse after the emergency room treatment of acute asthma. *N Engl J Med* 324 (1991): 788–94.

3. Terbutaline does come in an intravenous (IV) formulation that can be used in an intensive care unit for treatment of very severe asthma flare-ups.

4. Beam, W. R., Weiner, D. E., Martin, R. J. Timing of prednisone and

alterations of airways inflammation in nocturnal asthma. *Am Rev Respir Dis* 146 (1992): 1524–30.

5. Farber, H. J., Johnson, C., Beckerman, R. C. Young inner-city children visiting the emergency room for asthma: Risk factors and chronic care behaviors. *J Asthma* 35 (1998): 547–52.

6. Brunette, M. G., Lands, L., Thibodeau, L. P. Childhood asthma: Prevention of attacks with short-term corticosteroid treatment of upper-respiratory tract infection. *Pediatrics* 81 (1988): 624–69.

9. *Putting It All Together: How to Create an Asthma Self-Management Plan*

1. Farber, H. J., Smith-Wong, K., Nichols, L., Langham, B. Patients prefer simple, visual asthma self management plan forms. *Permanente Journal*, in press.

2. Available for free download at www.nhlbi.nih.gov/health/prof/lung/asthma/practgde.htm.

3. Greening, A. P., Ind, P. W., Northfield, M., Shaw, G. Added salmeterol versus higher-dose corticosteroid in asthma patients with symptoms on existing inhaled corticosteroid. *Lancet* 344 (1994): 219–24.

4. Evans, D. J., Taylor, D. A., Zetterstrom, O., Chung, K. F., O'Connor, B. J., Barnes, P. J. A comparison of low-dose inhaled budesonide plus theophylline and high-dose inhaled budesonide for moderate asthma. *N Engl J Med* 337 (1997): 1412–18.

5. Farber, H. J., Budson, D. A pediatric case of severe chronic interstitial lung disease presenting as spontaneous pneumothorax: Blame it on the birds. *Pediatric Asthma, Allergy, and Immunology* 14 (2000): 75–85.

10. *Finding the Right Doctor*

1. Farber, H. J., Johnson, C. Beckerman, R. C. Young inner-city children visiting the emergency room for asthma: Risk factors and chronic care behaviors. *J Asthma* 35 (1998): 547–52; Diaz, T., Sturm, T., Matte, T., Bindra, M., Lawler, K., Findley, S., Maylahn, C. Medication use among children with asthma in East Harlem. *Pediatrics* 105 (2000): 1188–93; Taylor, D. M., Auble, T. E., Calhoun, W. J., Mosesso, V. N., Jr. Current outpatient management of asthma shows poor compliance with international consensus guidelines. *Chest* 116 (1999): 1638–45.

2. Plaut, T. F. *Children with Asthma: A Manual for Parents*. Amherst, Mass.: Pedipress, Inc., 1995.

3. Lieu, T. A., Quesenberry, C. P., Jr., Capra, A. M., Sorel, M. E., Martin, K. E., Mendoza, G. R. Outpatient management practices associated with reduced risk of pediatric asthma hospitalization and emergency department visits. *Pediatrics* 100 (1997): 334–41; Finkelstein, J. A., Lozano, P., Farber, H. J., Streiff, K. A., Miroshnik, I., Lieu, T. A. Underuse of controller medications among Medicaid-insured asthma patients (abstract). *Pediatr Res* 47 (2000): 188A.

11. *Getting Your Health Plan On Board*

1. National Heart Lung and Blood Institute, *Data Fact Sheet: Asthma Statistics.* January 1999.

2. Finkelstein, J. A., Lozano, P., Farber, H. J., Streiff, K. A., Miroshnik, I., Lieu, T. A. Underuse of controller medications among Medicaid-insured asthma patients (abstract). *Pediatr Res* 47 (2000): 188A.

Lieu, T. A., Quesenberry, C. P., Sorel, M. E., Mendoza, G. R., Leong, A. B. Computer-based models to identify high-risk children with asthma. *Am J Respir Crit Care Med* 157 (1998): 1173–80.

3. Zeiger, R. S., Heller, S., Mellon, M. H., Wald, J., Falkoff, R., Schatz, M. Facilitated referral to asthma specialist reduces relapses in asthma emergency room visits. *J Allergy Clin Immunol* 87 (1991): 1160–68; Westley, C. R., Spiecher, B., Starr, L. Simons, P., Sanders, B., Marsh, W., Comer, C., Harvey, R. Cost-effectiveness of an allergy consultation in the management of asthma. *Allergy Asthma Proc* 18 (1997): 15–18; Doan, T., Grammer, L. C., Yarnold, P. R., Greenberger, P. A., Patterson, R. An intervention program to reduce the hospitalization cost of asthmatic patients requiring intubation. *Ann Allergy Asthma Immunol* 76 (1996): 513–58.

4. NIH, *National Asthma Education and Prevention Program Expert Panel Report 2: Guidelines for the Diagnosis and Management of Asthma.* Publication no. 97–4051 (April 1997). Available for download at http://www.nhlbi. nih.gov/nhlbi/lung/asthma/prof/asthgdln.htm.

12. *Choosing and Using Tools*

1. Wildhaber, J. H., Janssens, H. M., Piérart, F., Dore, N. D., Devadason, S. G, LeSouëf, P. N. High-percentage lung delivery in children from detergent-treated spacers. *Pediatr Pulmonol* 29 (2000): 389–93.

2. Turner, M. O., Patel, A., Ginsburg, S., FitzGerald, J. M. Bronchodilator delivery in acute airflow obstruction: A Meta-analysis. *Arch Intern Med* 157 (1997): 1736–44; Newhouse, M. T. Asthma therapy with aerosols: Are nebulizers obsolete? A continuing controversy. *J Pediatr* 135 (1999): 5–8.

14. *Infants and Toddlers*

1. Martinez, F. D., Wright, A. L., Taussig, L. M., Holberg, C. J., Halonen, M., Morgan, W. J., et al. Asthma and wheezing in the first six years of life. *N Engl J Med* 332 (1995): 133–38.

2. Agertoft, L., Pedersen S. Effects of long-term treatment with an inhaled corticosteroid on growth and pulmonary function in asthmatic children. *Respir Med* 88 (1994): 373–81.

3. For a list of diseases that can mimic asthma as well as criteria for the need to visit a specialist, see the National Heart Lung and Blood Institute. *Expert*

Panel Report 2: *Guidelines for the Diagnosis and Management of Asthma*, at
http://www.nhlbi.nih.gov/guidelines/asthma/asthgdln.htm.

16. *Asthma outside the Home*

1. Anto, J. M., Sunyer, J., Rodriguez-Roisin, R., Suarez-Cervera, M.,
Vazquez, L. Community outbreaks of asthma associated with inhalation of soy-
bean dust. *N Engl J Med* 320 (1989): 1097–102; White, M. C., Etzel, R. A.,
Olson, D. R., Goldstein, I. F. Reexamination of epidemic asthma in New
Orleans, Louisiana, in relation to the presence of soy at the harbor. *Am J Epi-
demiol* 145 (1997): 432–38.

2. Rosenlund, M., Bluhm, G. Health effects resulting from nitrogen dioxide
exposure in an indoor ice arena. *Arch Environ Health* 54 (1999): 52–57; Morgan, W. K. Zamboni disease: Pulmonary edema in an ice hockey player. *Arch
Intern Med* 155 (1995): 2479–80.

3. Rosenstreich, D. L., Eggleston, P., Kattan, M., Baker, D., Slavin, R. G.,
Gergen, P., et al. The role of cockroach allergy and exposure to cockroach allergen in causing morbidity among inner-city children with asthma. *N Engl J Med*
336 (1997): 1356–63.

4. Anto, J. M., Sunyer, J., Reed, C. E., Sabria, J., Martinez, F., Morell, F., et
al. Preventing asthma epidemics due to soybeans by dust-control measures. *N
Engl J Med* 329 (1993): 1760–63.

17. *Complementary and Alternative Treatments*

1. Field, T., Henteleff, T., Hernandez-Reif, M., Martinez, E., Mavunda, K.,
Kuhn, C., Schanberg, S. Children with asthma have improved pulmonary functions after massage therapy. *J Pediatr* 132 (1998): 854–88.

2. Balon, J., Aker, P. D., Crowther, E. R., Danielson, C., Cox, P. G.,
O'Shaughnessy, D., Walker, C, Goldsmith, C. H., Duku, E., Sears, M. R. A
comparison of active and simulated chiropractic manipulation as adjunctive
treatment for childhood asthma. *N Engl J Med* 339 (1998): 1013–20.

18. *The Future of Asthma Care*

1. Lindquist, M., Edwards, I. R. Risks of non-sedating antihistamines.
Lancet 349 (1997): 1322; DuBuske, I. M. Second-generation antihistamines:
The risk of ventricular arrhythmias. *Clin Ther* 21 (1999): 281–95.

2. Milgrom, H., Fick, R. B., Su, J. Q., Reimann, J. D., Bush, R. K., Watrous,
M. L., Metzger, W. J. Treatment of allergic asthma with monoclonal anti-IgE
antibody. *N Engl J Med* 341 (1999): 1966–73.

3. von Mutius, E., Martinez, F., Fritzsch, C., Nicolai, T., Roell, G., Thiemann, H. Prevalence of asthma and atopy in two areas of West and East Germany. *Am J Respir Crit Care Med* 149 (1994): 358–64.

4. Martinez, F. D., Wright, A. L., Taussig, L. M., Holberg, C. J., Halonen, M., Morgan, W. J., et al. Asthma and wheezing in the first six years of life. *N Engl J Med* 332 (1995): 133–38.

5. Ball, T. M., Castro-Rodriguez, J. A., Griffith, K. A., Holberg, C. J., Martinez, F. D., Wright, A. L. Siblings, day care attendance, and the risk of asthma and wheezing during childhood. *N Engl J Med* 343 (2000): 538–43; Illi, S., von Mutius, E., Bergmann, R., Lau, S., Niggermann, B., Wahn, U., et al. Upper respiratory tract infections in the first year of life and asthma in children up to the age of 7 years (abstract). *Am J Respir Crit Care Med* 161 (March 2000): A704.

6. Remes, S. T., Castro-Rodriguez, J. A., Holberg C. J., Martinez, F. D., Taussig, L., Wright, A. Pet exposure in infancy and wheeze and asthma in childhood (abstract). *Am J Respir Crit Care Med* 161 (March 2000): A704.

7. Braun-Fahrlander, C., Gassner, M., Grize, L., Neu, U., Sennhauser, E. H., Varonier, H. S., Vuille, J. C., Wuthrich, B. Prevalence of hay fever and allergic sensitization in farmer's children and their peers living in the same rural community. *Clin Exp Allergy* 29 (1999): 28–34.

8. Martinez, F. D., Holt, P. G. Role of microbial burden in aetiology of allergy and asthma. *Lancet* 354 (1999): 12–15.

19. Frequently Asked Questions

1. Agertoft, L., Pedersen, S. Effects of long-term treatment with an inhaled corticosteroid on growth and pulmonary function in asthmatic children. *Respir Med* 88 (1994): 373–81.

Appendixes

APPENDIX A: Daily Asthma Diary

_____ 'S DAILY ASTHMA DIARY

Date/time							
AM Peak Flow/Asthma Zone							
PM Peak Flow/Asthma Zone							
Preventive Medicine 1:							
Preventive Medicine 2:							
Quick Reliever:							
Oral Steroid:							
Other Medicine:							
Asthma Symptoms: Score as: 0=none, 1=little, 2=some, 3=bad							
Cough							
Wheeze							
Chest tightness							
Exercise problem							
Sleep problem							
Breathing rate							

Instructions for use of the Asthma Diary:

Peak Flows: Every day write down the peak flow rate and asthma zone (G for green, Y for yellow, R for red).

Medicines: Fill in the names of the medications you use. Then place a check mark each time a puff is taken.

Asthma Symptoms: Score the amount of cough, wheeze, chest tightness, exercise problem, and sleep problem in each day's box.

Breathing Rate: Count the number of breaths taken in 60 seconds when your child is at rest or asleep.

Be sure to make a note in the margins about any special circumstances or change in routine.

Average Peak Flow Rates for Children*

Height (inches)	Peak Flow (L/min)[†]	Height (inches)	Peak Flow (L/min)
43	147	55	307
44	160	56	320
45	173	57	334
47	187	58	347
46	200	59	36
48	214	60	373
49	227	61	387
50	240	62	400
51	254	63	413
52	267	64	427
53	280	65	440
54	293	66	454
		67	467

*Adapted from "Pulmonology" by R. S. McCurley, in G. K. Sibert, R. Iannone, eds. *The Harriet Lane Handbook*. 15th ed. (St. Louis: Mosby Inc., 2000).

[†]Liters per minute.

These average peak flow rates by height for children can give you an estimate of about where your child's peak flow should be. Note that most children are either above or below average. It is important for you to know your child's *personal best* peak flow, that is, the best measure of what is normal for *your* child.

Selected Asthma Resources

A quick search on asthma using any of the Internet search engines will turn up a wealth of sites. Some pay careful attention to providing accurate information. Others are not as attentive to keeping their information accurate or up to date. Information provided often reflects the prejudices of the owner or sponsor of a site. Below are several asthma information sources that have an established track record of providing quality information and resources on asthma.

Government Organizations

National Heart Lung and Blood Institute
http://www.nhlbi.nih.gov/health/index.htm
http://www.nhlbt.nih.gov/health/public/lung/index.htm#asthma

The National Heart Lung and Blood Institute is the section of the National Institutes of Health that deals with lung diseases. The advantage of its Web site is that it is not biased or supported by commercial interests. There is some excellent, objective asthma information here, some written for consumers, some for health professionals. You can start with the practical information for patients and the general public, then work your way over to the "For health care professionals" side.

You can download the "Practical Guide for Diagnosis and Management of Asthma." If you still have energy left, then download the "Guidelines for the Diagnosis and Management of Asthma: NAEPP Expert Panel Report 2." Get through this much and you will have a solid knowledge foundation about asthma.

On the lung information for patients and the general public there are links for some excellent asthma education materials targeted to schools and schoolchildren. There is an educational pamphlet entitled, "Asthma and Physical Activity in the Schools," an educational curriculum for grade schoolchildren, "Asthma Awareness," as well as checklists for "Asthma Friendly" school and day care centers.

The United States Environmental Protection Agency, Indoor Environments Division
http://www.epa.gov/iag/

The Indoor Environments Division of the U.S. Environmental Protection Agency coordinates research and develops and implements policies regarding the impact of indoor air pollutants on the general public. Their Web site has excellent information on controlling asthma triggers in the home, at school, and in the workplace. A particularly valuable resource is their *Indoor Air Quality (IAQ) Tools for School Kit*. It contains detailed information and practical suggestions to show schools how to improve their indoor air quality at little or no cost.

Professional Societies

Professional societies are supported by dues paid by their members. Most professional societies also receive a significant part of their funding from pharmaceutical companies, both from educational grants and as advertising.

The American Academy of Allergy, Asthma, and Immunology
http://www.aaaai.org/public/default.stm

The American Association of Allergy, Asthma, and Immunology is a professional society of allergists. Their Web site contains a large store of good information on asthma. They even have a "Just for Kids" section.

The National Allergy Bureau
http://www.aaaai.org/nab/default.stm
   The National Allergy Bureau (NAB) is the section of the American Academy of Allergy, Asthma and Immunology's Aeroallergen Network. This is the source that many news organizations use to obtain the pollen counts. You too can find out the pollen and mold spore counts in your area from their Web site or by calling 800-9-POLLEN.

Charitable Organizations

Most charitable organizations interested in asthma receive a portion of their funding from the pharmaceutical industry.

American Lung Association (ALA)
http://www.lungusa.org/asthma
   The American Lung Association is a charitable organization dedicated to promoting lung health. The ALA funds research, patient education programs, and sponsors asthma camps. The American Lung Association has developed an excellent asthma education curriculum ("Open Airways for Schools") for elementary school students. Asthma camps are an opportunity for children with asthma to have fun, to establish friendships with other children who have asthma, and, at the same time, learn about their own asthma.
   There is lots of excellent information about asthma available on the ALA Internet site. Call your local lung association for information on asthma, asthma camps, and other lung health–related activities in your area. The phone number is easy to remember: 800-LUNG-USA.

Asthma and Allergy Foundation of America
http://www.aafa.org/
   The Asthma and Allergy Foundation of America (AAFA) is dedicated to improving the quality of life for people with asthma and allergies through education, advocacy, and research. AAFA has multimedia asthma education materials available for sale and has developed an exciting new asthma education curriculum for teenagers ("Power Breathing"). AAFA runs asthma camps and asthma patient support groups at various locations around the country. Call 800-7-ASTHMA.

Allergy and Asthma Network/Mothers of Asthmatics
http://www.aanma.org/

An advocacy organization that publishes newsletters, information sheets, booklets, and books on a variety of subjects related to allergies and asthma. Mothers of Asthmatics has produced a couple of really nice booklets for young children, including "I'm a Meter Reader" and "So You Have Asthma Too." Phone: 800-878-4403.

Medical Centers

Medical centers make most of their money from patient care. Research and educational grants often provide a significant portion of their funding. Sources of these grants include government agencies, private philanthropies, as well as the pharmaceutical industry.

National Jewish Medical Center
http://www.nationaljewish.org

The National Jewish Medical Center built its reputation for excellence in research and treatment of lung diseases. They will provide many pamphlets about asthma and other lung diseases. By calling their Lung Line (800-222-LUNG), you can ask questions of a nurse free of charge.

Children's Hospital of Iowa
http://www.vh.org/Patients/IHB/Peds/Allergy/Asthma/AsthmaHome.
html

The Children's Hospital of Iowa has built a wonderful patient education Web site called the Virtual Children's Hospital. It has an excellent and comprehensive section on asthma that has been written and reviewed by their local asthma experts. Once you have read the section on asthma for patients, go on to the section written for health care providers at http://www.vh.org/Providers/ClinGuide/Asthma/Asthma.
html.

Kaiser Permanente
http://www.kaiserpermanente.org/index.html

Most Kaiser Permanente medical centers have health education centers where you can view, borrow, or purchase a variety of pamphlets, books, and videos on asthma. Asthma classes for children and adults are available for a small fee at most Kaiser Permanente medical centers. These resources are usually available to both members and nonmembers of the Kaiser Foundation Health Plan. Call the Kaiser Permanente medical center nearest you.

There is some good information about asthma available on the Kaiser Permanente Web site; however, you have to search for it. Use the keyword "asthma."

The text of a pamphlet on asthma, written by Harold Farber, M.D., is available at http://www.kaiserpermanente.org/locations/california/mod02/mod02-11.html.

You can purchase "Your Child and Asthma," a professionally produced video on asthma care for $4.95 plus tax, shipping, and handling. Call 800-556-9444 to order. Or you can view this video free of charge at most Kaiser Permanente health education centers.

Allergy Supply Houses

Allergy supply houses sell equipment useful for allergy control. Prices of materials may vary between suppliers, so it pays to shop around. Some items (such as allergen-proof mattress and pillow covers) have good evidence of effectiveness. Other items (like chemicals to kill dust mites) may not have good evidence supporting their utility. Some items (like allergen-proof vacuums) may vary widely in price, with some HEPA-filtered vacuums selling for under $200 and others selling for well over $1,000.

National Allergy Supply
http://www.natlallergy.com
National Allergy Supply sells a wide variety of allergy-control materials. They also have allergy control information available as pamphlets, videos, and on their Web site. Phone: 800-522-1448.

Allergy Control Products
http://www.allergycontrol.com/
Allergy Control Products sells a wide variety of allergy-control materials. Their information on allergen control is generally of good quality. Phone: 800-422-DUST.

Allergy Asthma Technology Limited
http://www.allergyasthmatech.com

Allergy Asthma Technology, Ltd., has a comprehensive selection of allergy products at competitive prices. The information in their catalog on allergen control is of good quality. Phone: 800-621-5545.

Gazoontite.com
http://www.gazoontite.com/

This is one of the newest entrants into the allergy supply arena. They have a wide variety of materials available; however, some items seem pricey. The German term "Gesundheit!" is intentionally misspelled as their name. Phone: 800-4MY-NOSE.

Pedipress
http://www.pedipress.com/

Pedipress is a private, for-profit company that markets the asthma tools and educational materials that have been developed by Thomas Plaut, M.D.

Dr. Plaut has an excellent asthma diary form in three colors. A children's book, *Winning Over Asthma*, explains facts about asthma through the experiences of a five-year-old boy. Phone: 800-611-6081.

Stop-Smoking Resources

Most health systems, including Kaiser Permanente, offer stop-smoking classes, as do many community centers and clinics.

The American Lung Association has a wealth of information on quitting smoking. They have just started an on-line stop smoking program. Find it at www.lungusa.org/ffs.

Call your **local lung association** to find out about stop-smoking resources in your community. You can reach them at 800-LUNG-USA.

The California Smokers Helpline sponsors over-the-phone stop-smoking programs. They can also give you information to help you quit smoking. Call them at 800-NO-BUTTS.

The American Cancer Society sponsors the Great American Smokeout each November. The ACS helps people learn about the health hazards of smoking and become successful ex-smokers. Look up their local chapter in your phone book or call their national office at 404-320-3333. Or find their information on smoking on the Web at http://www. cancer.org/tobacco/index.html.

The **American Heart Association** produces a variety of publications and audiovisual materials about the effects of smoking on the heart. The AHA has also developed a guidebook for incorporating a weight-control component into smoking cessation programs. Look up their local chapter in your phone book or call their national office at 214-373-6300.

The **Office of the Surgeon General** publishes excellent educational material on quitting smoking. Find them on the Web at http://www. surgeongeneral.gov/tobacco.

The **Agency for Health Care Research and Policy** offers excellent guides for quitting smoking as well as other health issues. Find them on the Web at http://www.ahrq.gov/consumer/index.html#smoking.

An excellent detailed pamphlet on quitting smoking published by the **National Cancer Institute** is available on the Internet at http://rex.nci. nih.gov/NCI Pub Interface/Clearing the Air/clearing.html.

Rating Health Plans

National Center for Quality Assurance (NCQA)
http://www.ncqa.org

The National Center for Quality Assurance (NCQA) is an independent, nonprofit organization whose mission is to evaluate and report on the quality of the nation's managed care organizations.

Using the NCQA site, you can easily create a "report card" that rates health plans available in your area. You can find ratings on many areas, including access and service, qualified providers, staying healthy, getting better, living with illness, and accreditation status. Look at it before choosing a health plan.

Index

About the Authors

HAROLD FARBER, M.D., a board-certified pediatric pulmonologist (specialist in the lung diseases of children), is assistant chief of pediatrics for Kaiser Permanente in the Napa and Solano counties of northern California. He serves as chair of the Continuing Medical Education Committee for the American Lung Association of the East Bay and as chair of the Community Health Committee for the Solano County Medical Society. He lives in Vallejo, California.

MICHAEL BOYETTE is a veteran medical journalist. His books include *The Attention Deficit Answer Book* (with Alan Wachtel, M.D.). He lives in Philadelphia, Pennsylvania.